The History of Medicine

Greek and Roman Medicine

Ian Dawson

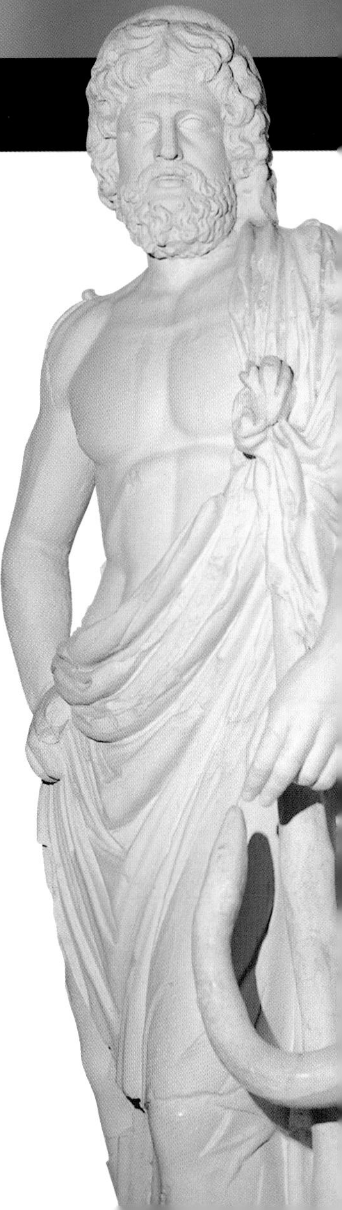

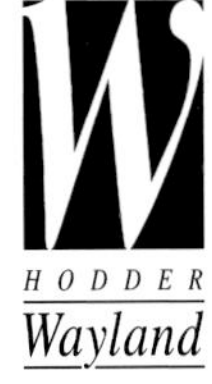

an imprint of Hodder Children's Books

First published in 2005 by Hodder Wayland,
an imprint of Hodder Children's Books

Series editor: Victoria Brooker
Editor: Deborah Fox
Inside design: Peta Morey
Cover design: Hodder Wayland
Picture research: Shelley Noronha, Glass Onion Pictures

British Library Cataloguing in Publication Data

Dawson, Ian, 1951 Aug. 25-
Greek & Roman medicine. - (History of medicine)
1.Medicine, Greek and Roman - Juvenile literature
I.Title
610.9'38

ISBN 0 7502 4512 3

Printed and bound in China

Hodder Children's Books
A division of Hodder Headline Limited
338 Euston Road, London NW1 3BH

Picture Acknowledgements. The author and publisher would like to thank the following for allowing their pictures to be reproduced in this publication: AKG Images: Erich Lessing, Archaeological Museum, Istanbul 11, Erich Lessing, Kunsthistorisches Museum, Vienna 24, 45; The Art Archive: Musée d'art et d'histoire Geneva/Dagli Orti 6, Jarrold Publishing 12, British Library 17, National Archaeological Museum Athens/Dagli Orti 23, Musée du Louvre Paris/Dagli Orti 25, Bibliothèque des Arts Décoratifs Paris/Dagli Orti 26, Archaeological Museum Naples/Dagli Orti 28, Bibliothèque des Arts Décoratifs Paris/Dagli Orti, 29, Dagli Orti 33, 48, 49, Archaeological Museum Ostia/Dagli Orti 36, Archaeological Museum Madrid/Dagli Orti 41, Museo Prenestino Palestrina/Dagli Orti 54, Anagni Cathedral Italy/Dagli Orti 59; Bridgeman Art Library (www.bridgeman.co.uk), Catacomb della Via Latina, Rome, Italy 14, Ecole Nationale Superieure des Beaux-Arts, Paris, France 19, Bibliotheque Municipale, Laon, France 35, New-York Historical Society, New York 57; CM DIXON title, 9, 10, 13, 21, 37, 39, 52, 55; Corbis: ED Eckstein, 15, Bettmann 18, Stephanie Colasanti 20, Bibliotheque Nationale de France 31; Mary Evans 42, 43; RGZM, Mainz 38; Robert Harding Picture Library: Robert Estall 46, Roy Rainford 8; Science Museum/Science & Society Picture Library 27, 56; www.segedunum.com © Brian Rootham 51; Topfoto/HIP/British Museum 34; Wellcome Library, London 4, 5, 22, 30, 40, 44; York Archaeological Trust 53

Contents

Chapter 1

The world of the Greeks

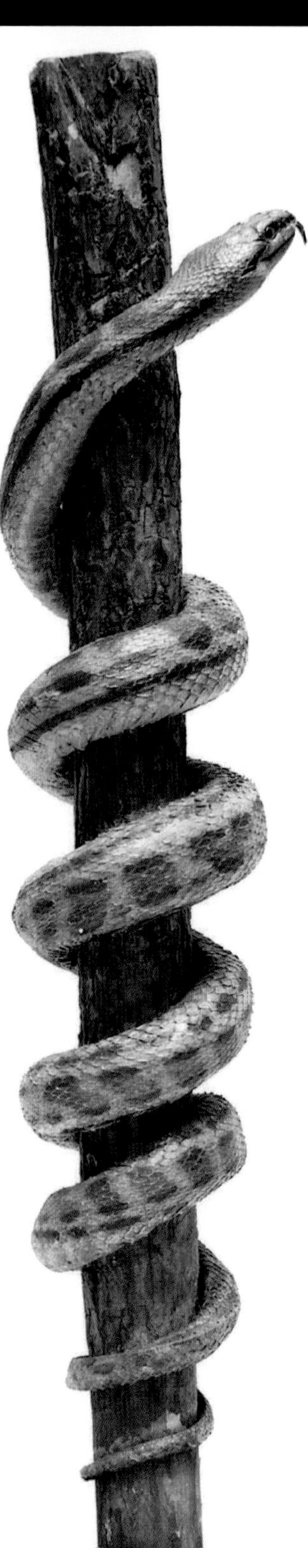

The importance of Greek and Roman medicine

Greek and Roman doctors played a crucial role in the history of medicine. The greatest of them, Hippocrates of Greece, was known for centuries as the 'Father of Medicine' and his Roman successor, Claudius Galen, as the 'Prince of Physicians'. Their treatments and ideas were followed for well over a thousand years. All medical students read their books and no-one dared to suggest that any of their ideas or discoveries were wrong. It was not until the sixteenth century, at the time of the European Renaissance, that doctors began to challenge their ideas. Even then, the first criticisms of Hippocrates and Galen were met with gasps of outrage. It was their long-lasting impact on medicine that makes the medical developments of Greece and Rome so significant.

Earlier medical ideas

The Greeks and the Romans were not the first peoples to develop medical treatments and theories. Prehistoric people learned to use herbs and plants to ease pain and counter infections. By trial and error, they found ways to mend broken limbs. They believed that their gods caused diseases and cured them, if people said the right prayers.

The first peoples to live in towns also developed their medical knowledge. In Egypt, around 2000 BCE, there were doctors who specialized in treating different ailments, such as eye diseases. The Egyptians also identified the major organs in the body – the heart, lungs and brain – although they did not understand exactly what part they played in keeping people healthy. They also used many successful herbal treatments.

Asclepios, the Greek god of healing, was often portrayed holding a staff with a snake wrapped around it. The staff has been used as a badge by many modern medical organizations, creating a link between the medicine of today and the medicine of the Ancient Greeks.

Why Hippocrates is known as the 'Father of Medicine'

- Doctors continued to believe in his theory on the cause of illness for 2000 years.
- The first large collection of medical texts is known as the 'Hippocratic Collection'.
- His advice on how to observe and examine patients is still followed today.
- He insisted that doctors should keep careful notes of all their cases.
- He understood that many herbs and plants were good medicines, such as extract of willow bark, which he recommended for women during childbirth because it is an effective means of pain relief.
- Doctors today agree with his advice on staying healthy through exercise and diet.

A queue to see the doctor! A Greek doctor takes blood from a patient's arm while other patients wait their turn. This scene was painted on a vase *c.* 470 BCE.

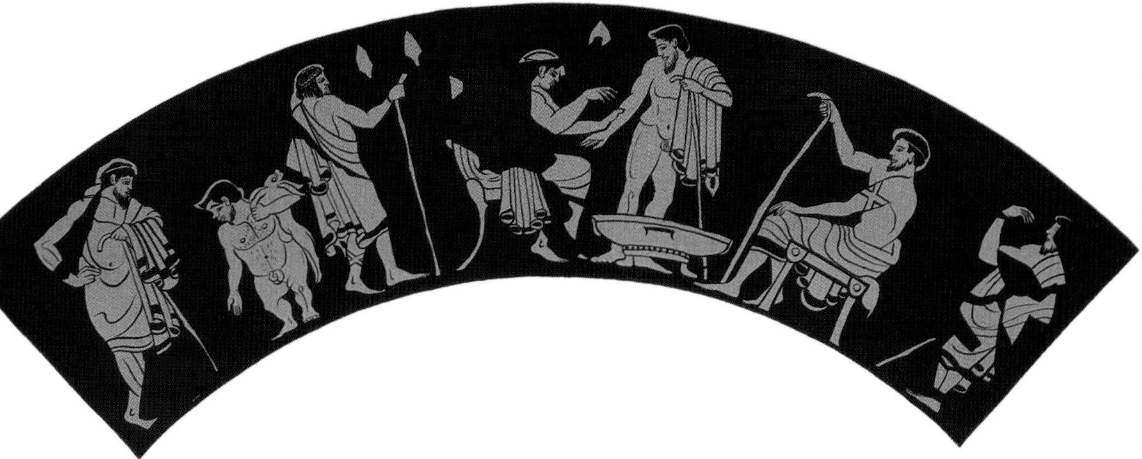

The Greeks borrowed ideas from the Egyptians on the use of herbal medicines, but they developed their own ideas about why people became ill and how to treat sickness. The Greeks' medical methods developed because of their lifestyle and the skills they had. To understand Greek medicine we have to understand some of the key features of the way the Greeks lived.

The Greek empire

Between 1500 BCE and 500 BCE, people from the area we now call Greece spread out all over the eastern Mediterranean. The Greeks were successful soldiers, conquering other peoples, including those in the Egyptian empire. The greatest Greek soldier of all was Alexander the Great, who was born in Macedonia in 356 BCE. Alexander became king, aged just twenty, when his father, Philip of Macedon, was murdered. In just thirteen years, Alexander won a huge empire that reached the borders of India and China, but, at the age of just 33, he died of fever. In his short life, he spread Greek ideas throughout the lands he conquered and founded many cities, including Alexandria in northern Egypt. It was to become the greatest centre for medical learning in the Greek and Roman worlds.

Although we talk about the Greek empire, for long periods there was no overall Greek government. Instead, the Greek empire was made up of independent cities such as Athens, Sparta and Corinth. In the fifth century BCE, Athens became the most powerful city state, thanks to her strong army and navy and her wealth from the mining of silver.

Alexander the Great astride his favourite horse, Bucephalus.

The Trojan War

The legendary Trojan War took place in about 1250 BCE. Hundreds of years later, the story of the Greek attack on the city of Troy was retold by the Greek writer Homer in his epic poem *The Iliad* (*Ilium* was the Greek name for Troy). According to Homer, the Greeks, led by the brothers Agamemnon and Menelaus, attacked Troy to win back Helen, the wife of Menelaus, who had run off with Paris, prince of Troy. *The Iliad* is full of battle scenes that provide us with evidence on how Greek surgeons treated wounds.

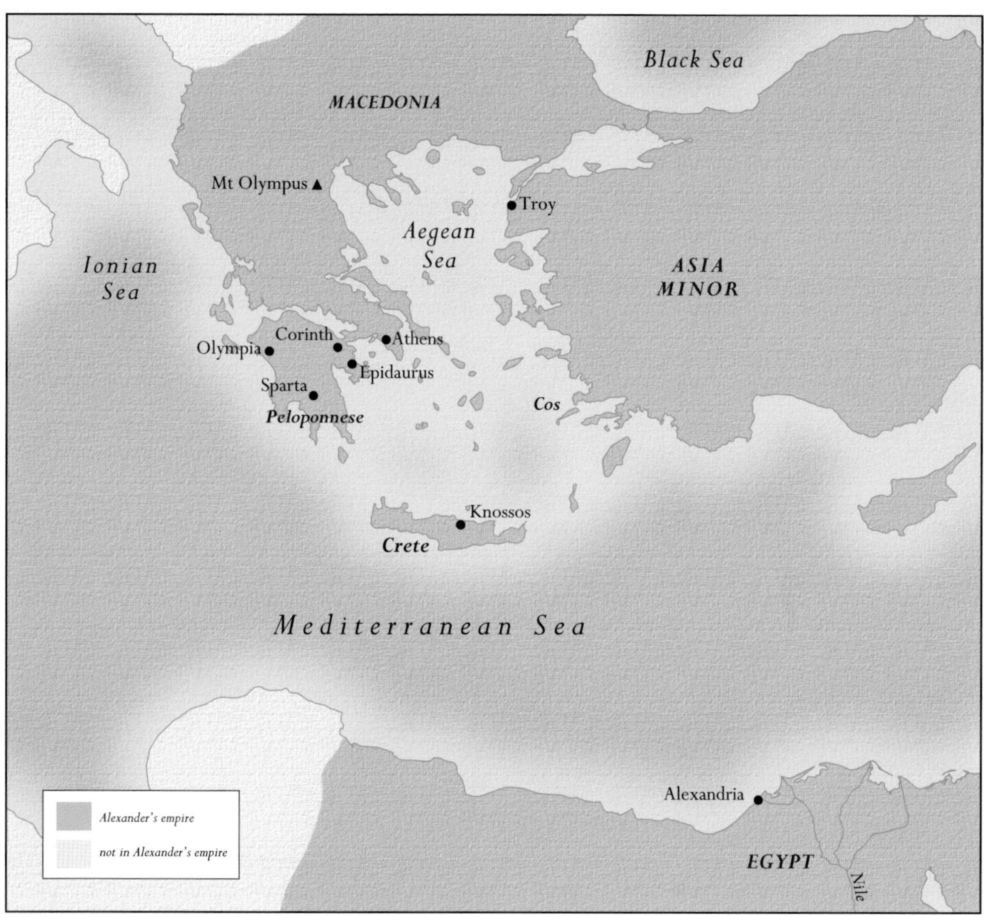

This map shows the major cities and sites in Ancient Greece and the extent of Alexander's empire *c.* 330 BCE. It stretched eastwards to the borders of India.

The city states were often ruled by small groups of men (called 'oligarchies') but, from 508 BCE, the laws of Athens were decided by the votes of male citizens at special meetings. This was the first example in history of democracy, or 'rule by the people'. Women, slaves and foreigners, however, were not allowed to vote.

The Greeks grew rich from farming, trade and mining precious metals. They also owned many slaves they had captured in wars. They spent their money on jewellery, decorated pottery, and armour and weapons made from the finest bronze and iron. They also built grand public buildings such as temples and theatres. Wealth provided them with time to practise athletic skills and improve their fitness. Their wealth, trade, craftsmanship and enthusiasm for athletics had a significant influence on their medical ideas and treatments.

Chapter 2

How did the god Asclepios help the sick?

The Greeks and their gods

Many of the most splendid buildings in Greece were the temples dedicated to the gods. Gods were central to the life of Ancient Greece. They were so important that the Athenians built their temples on the most important and dramatic site in the city. This was the Acropolis, the Greek term for 'high city', which stood on a rocky hill, overlooking Athens.

It is not surprising that the Greeks believed the gods were responsible for many illnesses when they played such a large part in Greek life. The epic poem *The Iliad* begins with a plague sent by the god Apollo as a punishment, because the Greeks had mistreated one of his priests. When Athens was hit by a terrible plague in 430–427 BCE, the people prayed to the gods to end the deaths and suffering.

The god of healing

By 400 BCE the god chiefly linked to medicine and healing was Asclepios. There were two different legends about him. One said that the real Asclepios had been a warrior chief, who was exceptionally skilful at healing

The Parthenon, on the Acropolis in Athens. The Parthenon is the main temple of the goddess Athene and was built from white marble in 447–438 BCE.

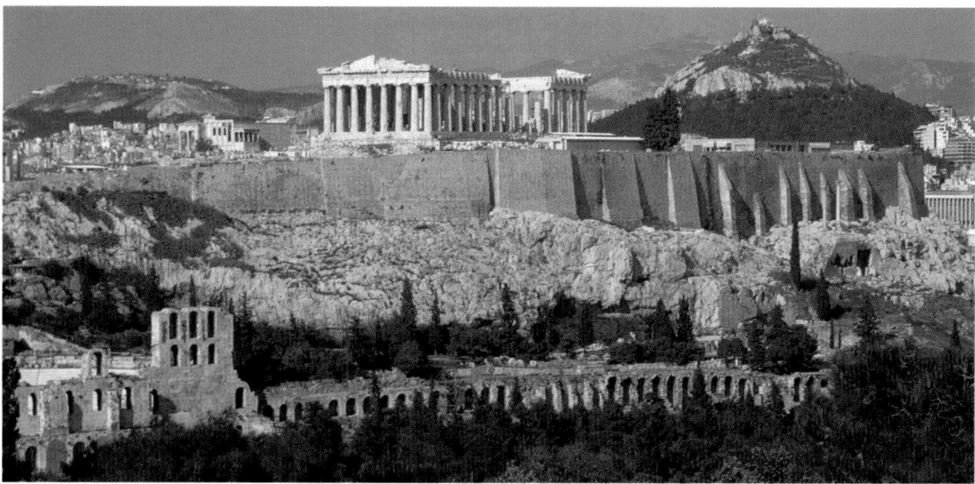

The gods of Ancient Greece

The Greeks believed the gods lived on Mount Olympus. The most important Greek gods were:

Zeus, the king of the gods
Hera, wife of Zeus and goddess of women
Poseidon, god of the sea
Demeter, goddess of grain who controlled the seasons and made all living things grow
Apollo, god of the sun and music
Aphrodite, goddess of love and beauty
Artemis, the huntress, protector of women and children
Pluto, god of the underworld
Athene, goddess of wisdom and war
Asclepios, the god of medicine and healing

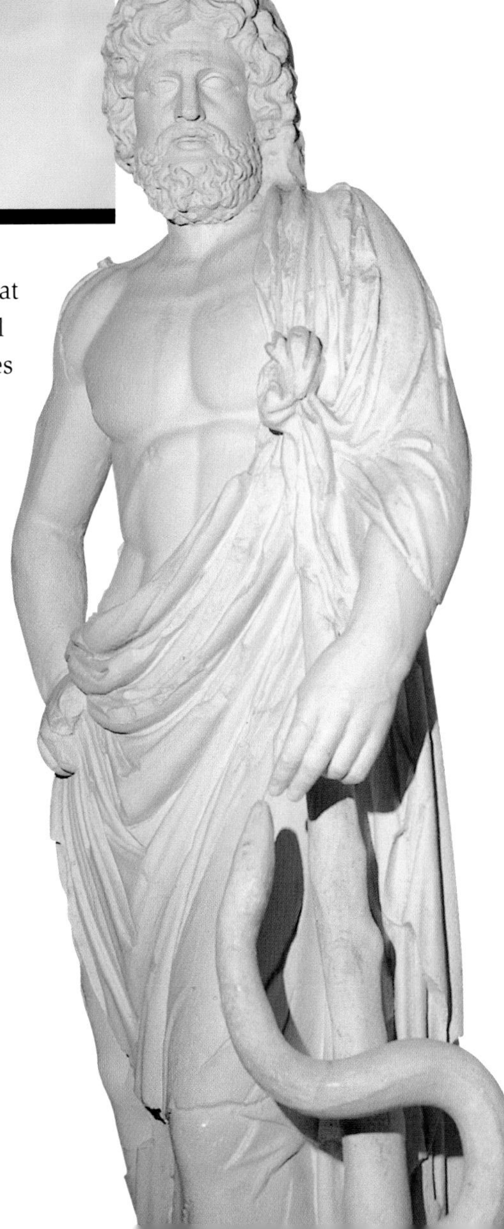
A statue of Asclepios, the god of medicine and healing, which stood at Epidaurus.

wounds. The other, more romantically, said that he was the son of the god Apollo and a mortal mother and that he was taught herbal remedies by Chiron the centaur, half man, half horse. We can never know whether there was a real healer called Asclepios, but we do know that Asclepios the god became very popular throughout Greece. By the third century BCE, temples called *Asclepeia* were built in every Greek town. They were places the sick could go in order to be healed by Asclepios.

The poet, Pindar, wrote of Asclepios:

"They came to him with ulcers the flesh had grown, or their
Limbs mangled with the grey bronze, or bruised
With the stone flung from afar,
Or the body stormed with summer fever, or chill, and he
Released each man and led him
From his individual grief."

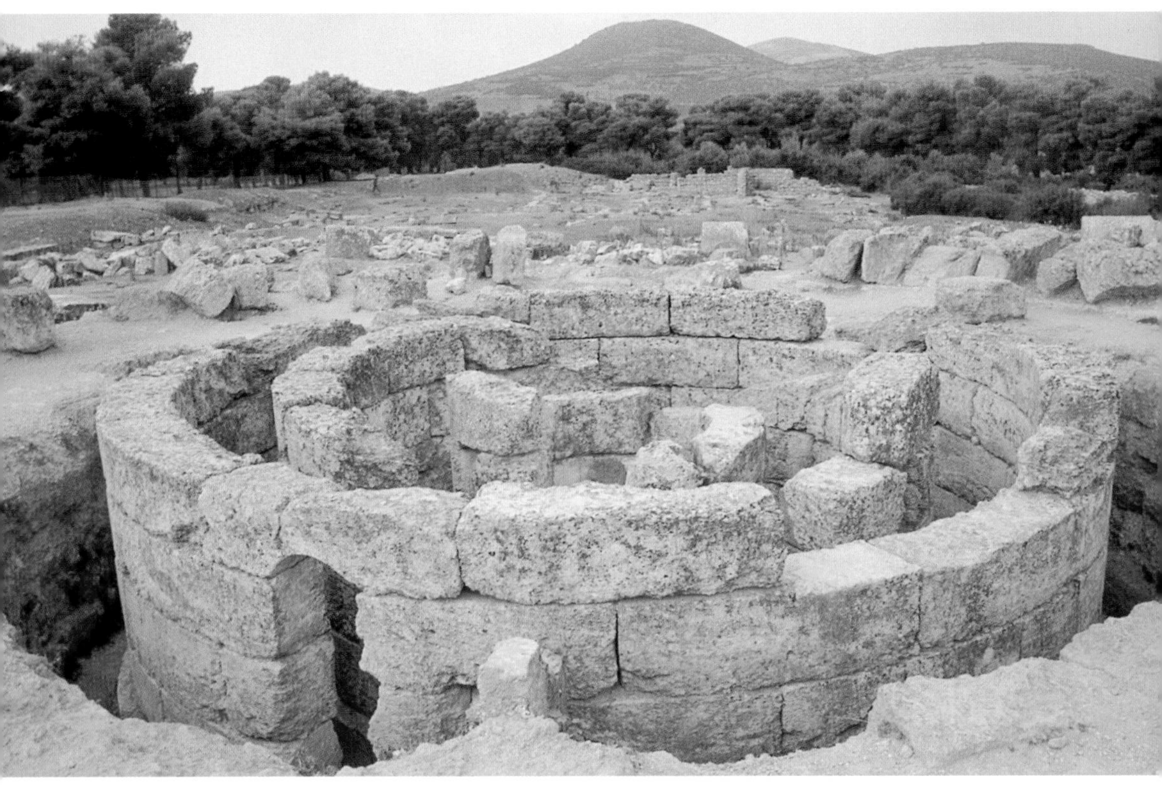

The remains of the *Asclepion* at Epidaurus, the largest in Greece, which contained baths, a gymnasium, an athletics stadium and even a theatre that seated an audience of 14,000. In the foreground is the *tholos*, a circular building where, it has been suggested, the sacred snakes were kept.

At the *Asclepion*

An *Asclepion* was not just a temple, it was similar to a modern health resort. The smallest *Asclepeia* contained a temple, the *abaton* (the long hall where the patients slept), and areas for walking and sitting quietly. However, some were much larger, such as the *Asclepion* at Epidaurus.

Men, women and children visited the *Asclepeia* with the strong hope that their illnesses would be cured by the god Asclepios. When they arrived, they were greeted by the temple priests and taken to the temple. There, on the altar, they put their gifts (such as cakes and honey) for Asclepios.

The priests at the *Asclepeia* were doctors as well as religious men. They encouraged the sick to take exercise and to cleanse themselves in the baths. The visitors also built up their strength by eating regular meals and they had time for plenty of rest and time for prayer. Some visitors stayed for weeks or even months.

Visions of Asclepios

At night, the sick slept in the hall. That was where they believed that the god Asclepios came to them and cured them. Today we would say that the cures were the work of the priests and that people simply dreamed that Asclepios had cured them, but writings show that the Greeks believed that Asclepios himself had been their healer. In his play *Plutus*, the writer Aristophanes (450–385 BCE) wrote a scene set in an *abaton*. The audience would have believed the following description was exactly what happened:

"The god Asclepios went round with calm and quiet steps to every patient looking at his disease. Then a servant placed a stone pestle and mortar and a medicine chest by his side. First the god wiped Plutus' head, then with a cloth of clean linen he wiped his eyelids a number of times. Next Panacea covered his face and head with a scarlet drape. The god whistled and two huge serpents appeared. They crept under the scarlet cloth and licked his eyelids. Then Plutus sat up and he could see again, but the god, his helpers and the serpents had vanished."

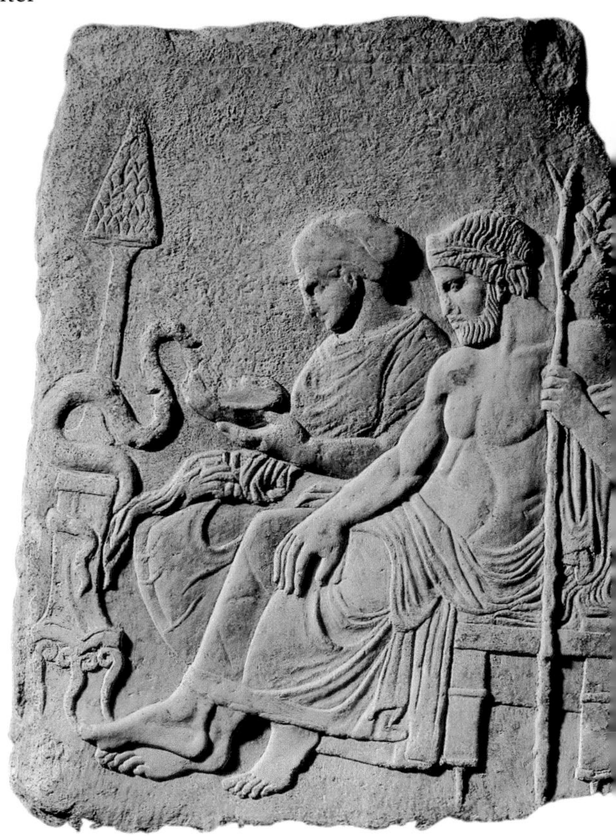

A carving of Asclepios and his daughter Hygeia, who is feeding the god's snake. Snakes became symbols of health because they could shed their skins, appearing younger and healthier. Harmless snakes were kept at *Asclepeia* and were left in the *abaton* overnight while patients slept.

Hygeia and Panacea

According to Greek legends, two of Asclepios' daughters – Hygeia and Panacea – were closely involved in healing patients. Their names are still part of our everyday vocabulary. Hygeia is remembered in words like 'hygiene', which means keeping clean to protect yourself from disease. Today a 'panacea' is a remedy that will cure all diseases and health problems.

Did the treatments at the *Asclepeia* work?

The evidence from the sites certainly suggests that people thought the treatments worked. Like the Egyptians before them, the Greeks believed that many illnesses had supernatural causes and cures. However, the evidence also shows that the priests were very practical healers. They took great care in cleaning the parts of the body that were affected.

There were over one hundred temples of Asclepios and the priests probably shared their experience and built up considerable knowledge of effective treatments. The temple priests also carried out simple surgery, probably while the patient was in a drug-induced sleep. One operation for which we have written evidence is the removal of fragments of a spearhead from a victim's cheek.

A carving showing Asclepios treating a patient. You can see the god's serpent taking part in the cure. It was believed that the serpent could cure blindness by licking the patients' eyelids.

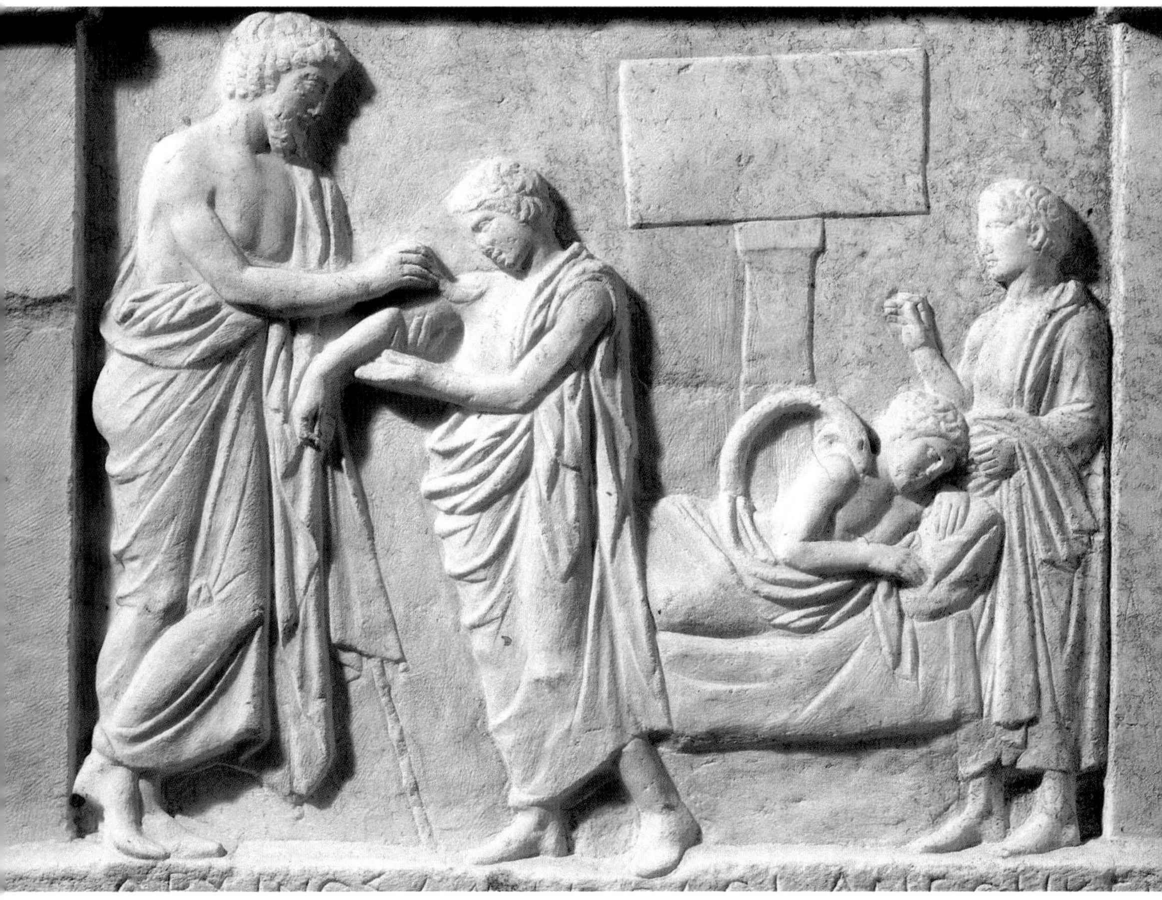

Votive stones

Grateful patients offered their thanks to Asclepios by paying for votive stones and dedicating them to the god. Archaeologists have discovered votive stones carved in the shape of the affected part of the body, such as an arm, a leg or an eye. Some have inscriptions describing the ailment and the cure and giving thanks to Asclepios. Some record recoveries from serious health problems such as a stomach abscess, and even complete paralysis.

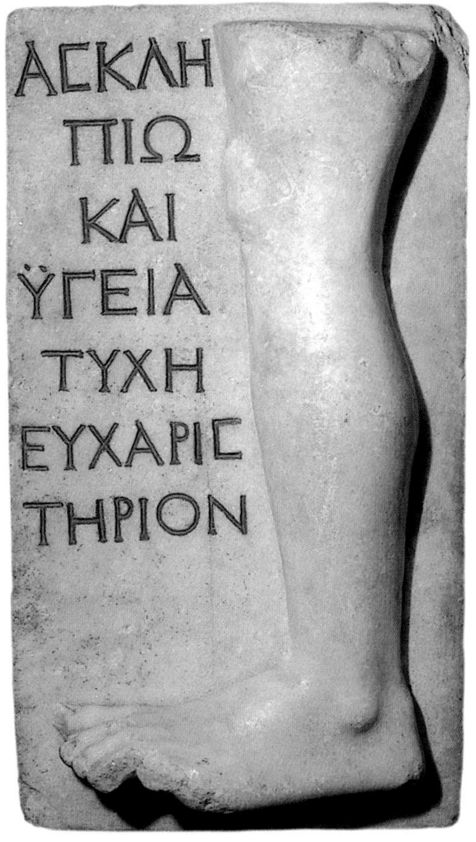

A votive stone excavated from an *Asclepion*. This larger than life-size stone suggests that the patient was extremely grateful for the treatment. The inscription honours Asclepios and his daughter Hygeia.

A lasting belief

The temples of Asclepios remained a central part of Greek medicine until about 300 BCE. They were one of the many medical ideas that the Romans borrowed from the Greeks. Even when Greek doctors developed new theories about illnesses having natural causes and cures, people still believed that they could be cured at the temples. The two approaches, supernatural and natural, existed side by side. This is not altogether surprising. Although the temple priests appeared to depend on supernatural appearances by the god Asclepios, they actually used a wide range of natural treatments, which they had developed through long experience.

Offerings to the god

One votive stone discovered at an *Asclepion* has the following inscription:

Agestratos was unable to sleep on account of headaches. As soon as he came to the abaton *he fell asleep and had a dream. He thought that the god cured him of his headache and, making him stand up, taught him wrestling. The next day he departed cured, and after a short time he competed at the Nemean games and was victor at wrestling.*

Chapter 3

What were the Greeks' new medical ideas?

Lovers of knowledge

The Greeks did not develop new medical ideas just by chance or because of a few brilliant individuals. They developed new ideas because many men were wealthy and did not need to spend all their time working as farmers or merchants. They used their time to study, to read and to learn more about the world around them. Athens was the home of many philosophers – a Greek word that means 'lovers of knowledge'. Great philosophers such as Socrates, Aristotle and Plato investigated politics, mathematics, astronomy and other sciences.

Philosophers asked questions about the origins of the world and of people. They looked for natural, logical answers to their scientific questions and did not simply accept the answer, "it was the gods". For example, Anaximander, who lived in about 560 BCE, argued that

A Roman painting from the fourth century CE, believed to show the Greek philosopher Aristotle instructing his students in anatomy.

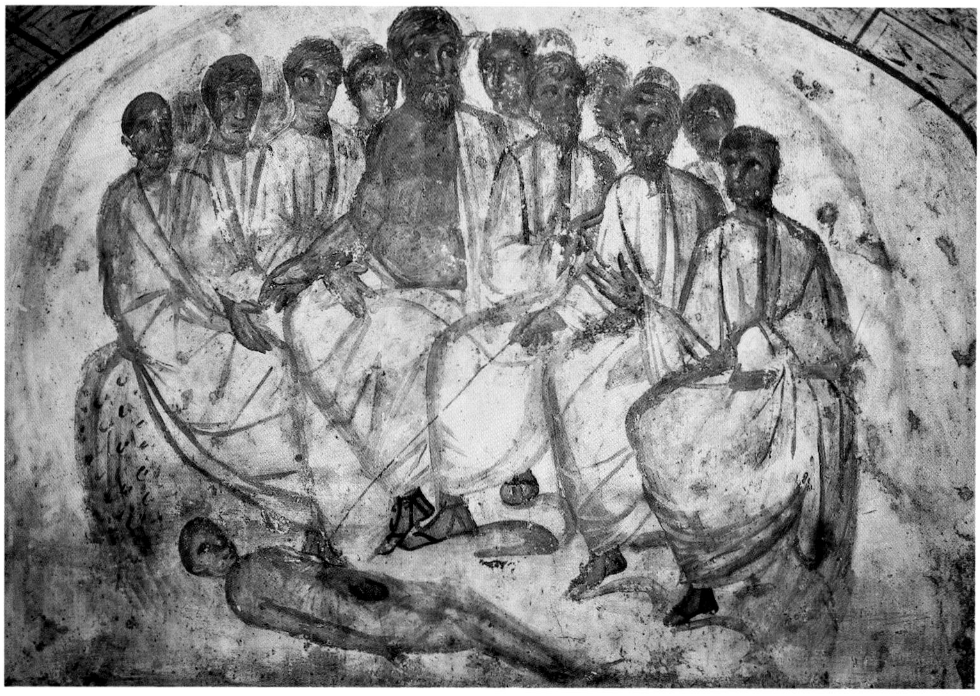

The Hippocratic Collection

The main evidence we have on Greek medicine comes from the many books written and collected by Greek doctors and scientists. These books are known as the 'Hippocratic Collection', but they were not all written by Hippocrates. They were written, re-written and re-organized by many writers over time and they were collected together in Alexandria in the third century BCE. The Collection consists of around 60 books with titles such as *A Programme for Health*, *On Epidemics*, *On Fractures* and *On the Treatment of Acute Diseases*.

thunder did not echo round the sky because the god Zeus was angry. He thought it was a natural phenomenon, caused by air becoming trapped in a cloud and bursting out with great force.

Who was Hippocrates?

Some philosophers turned their attention to medicine, to questions such as, "Why do people become ill?" The philosopher associated with the most important developments in medicine was Hippocrates, the most famous name in medical history. Despite his fame, we know very little about him at all. Legend says that he was born on the island of Cos *c.* 470 BCE and that he worked as a doctor and trained other doctors until he died nearly a hundred years later. Plato does, in fact, mention in one of his books a famous doctor called Hippocrates who was living around 430 BCE, but these are the only details we have about a man who was revered by doctors for the next 2000 years.

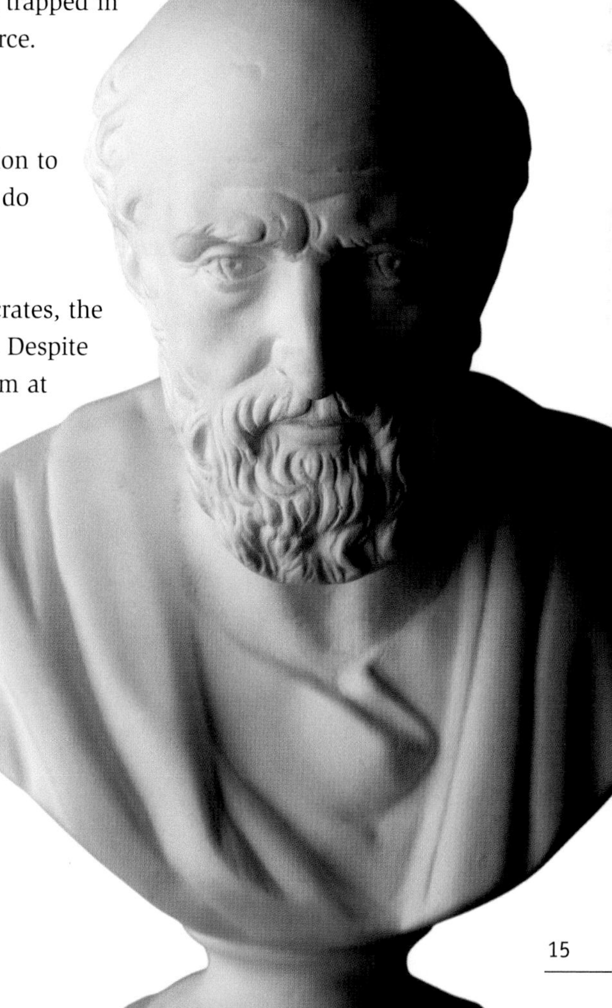

A bust of Hippocrates, by an unknown Greek sculptor.

The theory of the Four Humours

The most important idea associated with Hippocrates was the theory of the Four Humours. This was the Greeks' answer to the most important question in medicine ... "Why do people become ill?" Instead of blaming the gods, Greek doctors said that there was a natural, rational cause for illness. They believed that the body contained four important liquids, which they called humours. People stayed healthy while the humours were in balance but fell ill if they became unbalanced, with too much of one humour or too little of another.

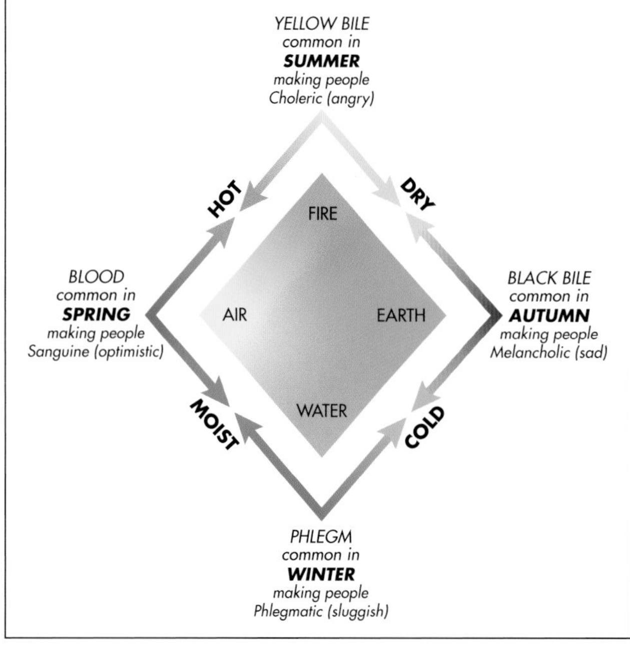

This diagram shows how the Four Humours were linked to the four elements and to the seasons.

This theory grew out of the work of Greek philosophers who wanted to understand what the world and its plants, animals and people were made of. They identified four basic elements in all things – air, fire, earth and water. These four elements became linked to the Four Humours and to the seasons as you can see from the illustration.

The humours were linked to illness because doctors observed and identified them when people were sick. Doctors witnessed phlegm, yellow bile and black bile when people vomited, and phlegm when a patient sneezed or had a cold. They saw blood when people had nosebleeds or their faces were flushed with a temperature.

Careful observation also linked the humours and the elements to the seasons. Doctors noted that people were often ill in winter with sneezes and runny noses. This showed they had too much phlegm, the humour linked to the element water, which was cold and moist – like winter!

The whole theory fitted together so perfectly that it was almost impossible to prove that it was wrong. It was not until the seventeenth and eighteenth centuries that the theory was strongly questioned and it was not until the mid-nineteenth century, with the help of microscopes and other scientific equipment, that Louis Pasteur and Robert Koch were able to prove that bacteria are the real causes of diseases. They finally disproved the theory of the Four Humours.

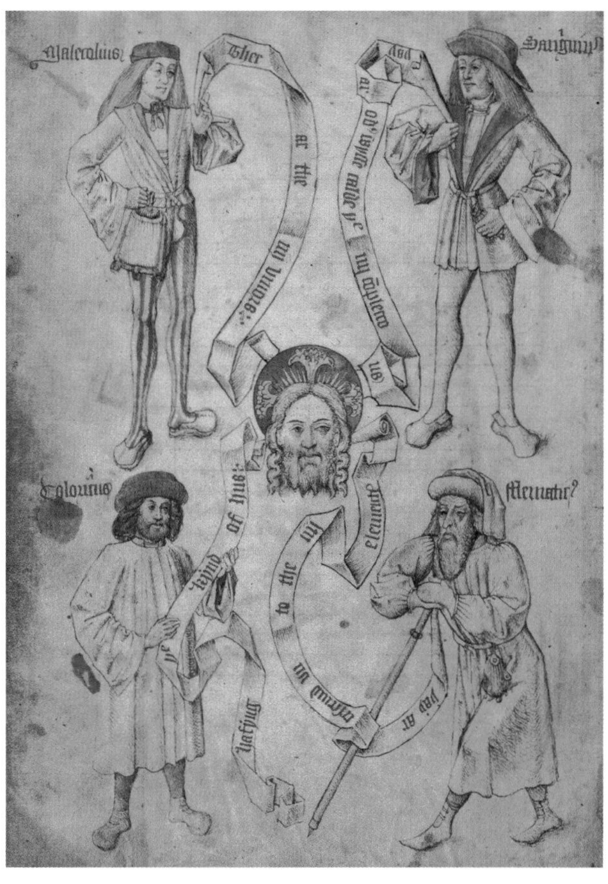

This illustration dates from 1500 CE and shows the four temperaments linked to the humours. The figures are (clockwise from the top right): the sanguine man, the phlegmatic, the choleric and the melancholic.

How to stay healthy

This quotation is from *On the Constitution of Man*, a book in the Hippocratic Collection:

Man's body ... has blood, phlegm, yellow bile and melancholy (black) bile. These make up his parts and through them he feels illness or enjoys health. When all these elements are truly balanced and mingled, he feels the most perfect health. Illness occurs when one of these humours is in excess, or is lessened in amount or is entirely thrown out of the body.

New discoveries about the human body

Greek doctors did not just develop theories about the cause of disease but also investigated the workings of the body. Aristotle (384–322 BCE), one of the greatest of all philosophers, recommended that doctors dissect animals in order to build up their understanding of the body. Aristotle dissected the eggs of animals and observed the embryos. He believed the heartbeat was the first sign of life. He said that the heart was the most important organ in the body, driving all the other parts, including the brain.

This nineteenth-century engraving gives an impression of what the great library at Alexandria might have looked like.

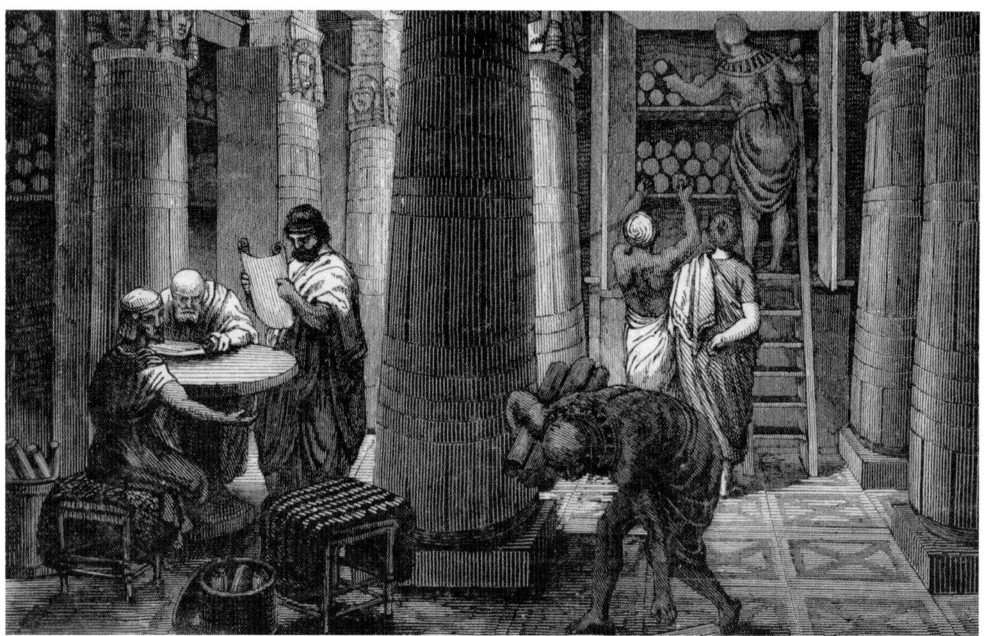

The great library at Alexandria

At Alexandria, the Greeks built a university and library that aimed to collect copies of all the books in the world. It was said to contain 700,000 books. Ships docking at Alexandria were searched and any books on board were taken to the library to be copied. Amongst the thousands of books was a collection of medical books from India, China and Mesopotamia, as well as titles by Hippocrates and other Greek writers. The library became the greatest centre of medical learning in the ancient world, attracting medical students from all around the Mediterranean until the eighth century CE, long after the fall of the Roman Empire.

However, dissection of human bodies was illegal in Greece, so it was difficult for doctors to develop detailed, accurate knowledge of anatomy (the structure of the body) and physiology (how the body works). Human dissection was allowed in Alexandria in Egypt and two physicians working there, Herophilus and Erasistratus, made important discoveries thanks to their careful dissections of human bodies.

Herophilus, who lived *c.* 335–280 BCE, discovered from dissecting human bodies that the brain, not the heart, controls the workings of the body. He also identified parts of the stomach. Erasistratus (*c.* 330–255 BCE) made detailed examinations of the brain too and also noted that the heart contained what seemed to be one-way valves. This made him wonder whether the heart was a pump, pumping air and blood around the body. It wasn't until the 1600s that William Harvey, an English scientist, proved that the heart pumps blood around the body.

One of the main reasons why it took so long to make other major discoveries was that, by about 200 BCE, human dissection was banned in Alexandria too. Scientists and doctors did not have the opportunity to undertake regular human dissections again, anywhere in Europe, until the sixteenth and seventeenth centuries – nearly two thousand years after the era of Herophilus and Erasistratus.

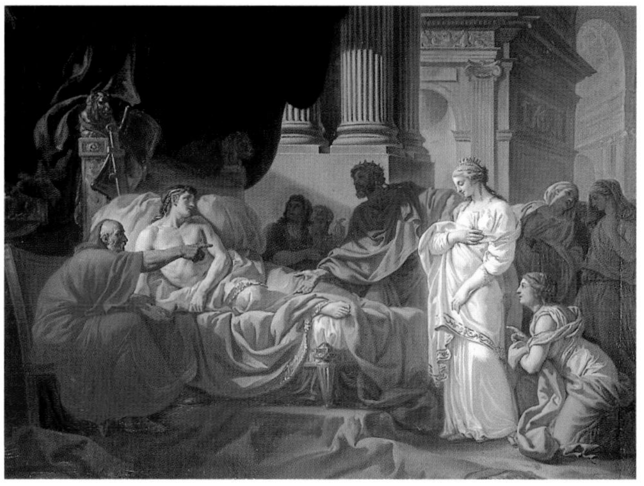

An eighteenth-century painting by Jacques David shows Erasistratus diagnosing that a king's son is suffering from love-sickness.

Chapter 4

How did Greek doctors try to heal the sick?

Who could you go to if you were ill?

If you had lived in a Greek city and had a little money to spare, you would have had a choice of healers. You could have chosen from a holy man, who would have provided you with prayers, a folk healer, with his charms and amulets, a woman healer with her well-tried herbal remedies, or a physician, one of the followers of Hippocrates, who would have asked you questions to arrive at his diagnosis. Some cities employed a city-physician to treat the local people, although they probably still had to pay a fee.

The tree on the island of Cos where legend says that Hippocrates sat and taught students about medicine. Under the tree is an old sarcophagus (a stone tomb) which was converted into a fountain.

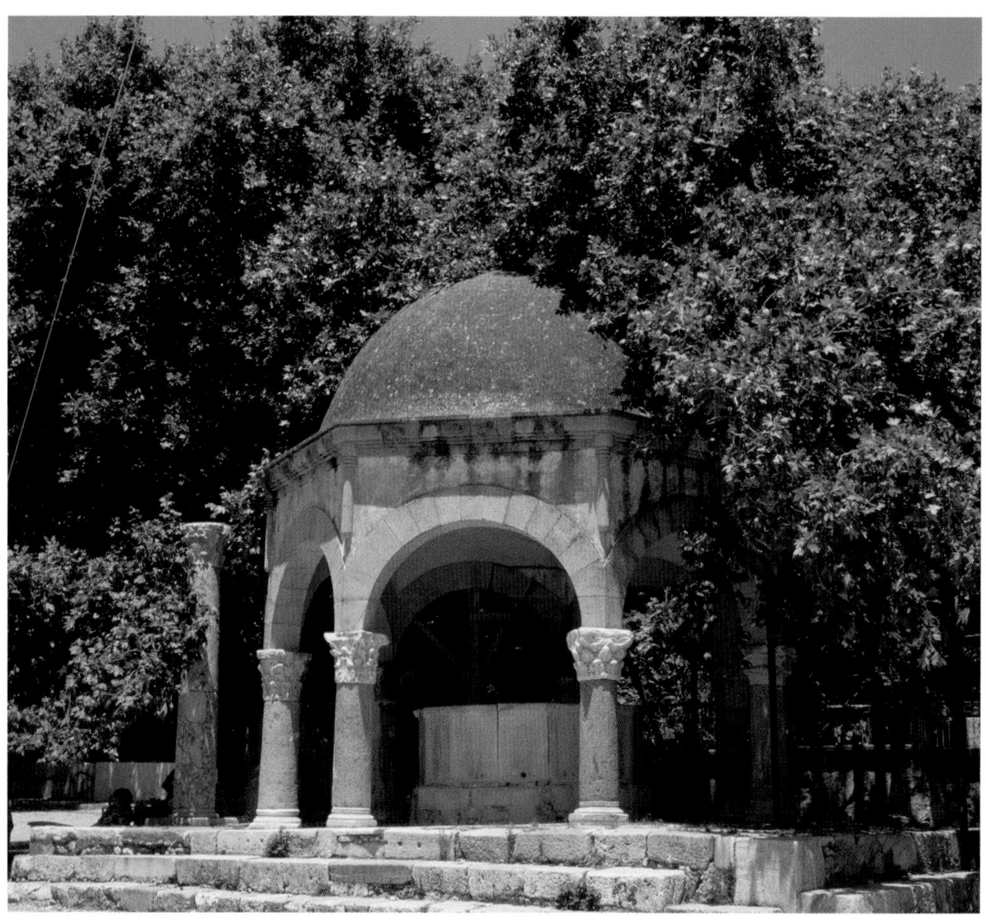

The physicians usually trained for several years as apprentices to another doctor, often their father or uncle. They would have studied the books in the Hippocratic Collection and a few – very few indeed – would have been to Alexandria or other cities to learn more about medicine. These physicians developed a series of promises to their patients, known as the 'Hippocratic Oath' (see below). The oath probably came about as a way of showing the physicians' high standards of knowledge and care and that they were superior to other healers.

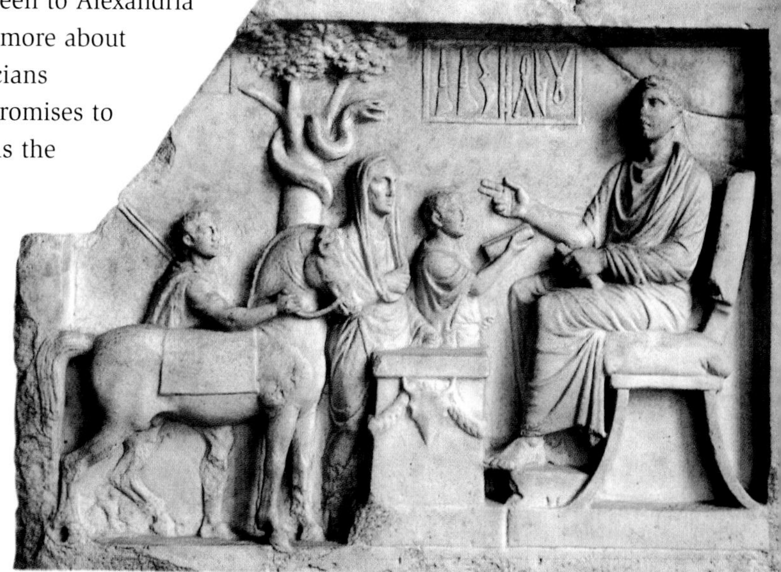

A Greek doctor and his patients. The serpent of Asclepios, the god of medicine, is keeping watch from the tree.

Women and medicine

We do not have as much evidence about medicine in the home as we do about the work of famous physicians. However, the few writings and carvings that remain suggest that when ordinary people fell ill, they turned to their mothers or wives for treatment. Women passed remedies, such as herbal cures, down through families. When a midwife was needed, older women with experience of childbirth were called in.

Extracts from the Hippocratic Oath

I swear by Apollo, the healer, by Asclepios, by Health and all the powers of healing ... that I may keep this Oath to the best of my ability and judgement.
I will use my power to help the sick to the best of my ability and judgement.
I will not give poison to anyone if I am asked, nor will I suggest any such thing.
Whatever I see or hear, professionally or privately, which ought not to be divulged, I will keep secret and tell no one.

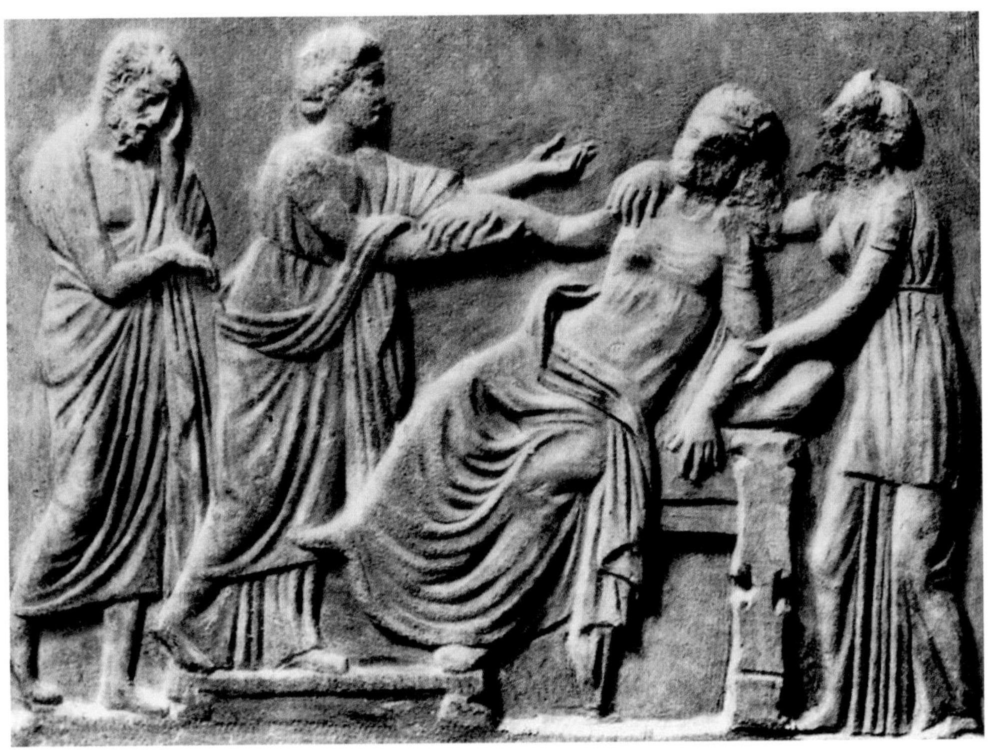

This plaque, dating from 350 BCE, shows a woman about to give birth. The woman's husband on the left looks worried and the midwife in the centre seems to be pleading. Many births must have caused great anxiety for the safety of mother and baby.

One of the first women doctors

Despite their everyday experience of treatments, remedies and childbirth, women were not allowed to learn the science of medicine. Officially they could not call themselves doctors or midwives because women were not allowed to play any part in public life in Greece.

However, the Greek writer Hyginus tells the story of a girl called Hagnodice who was determined to become a doctor. Hagnodice cut her hair short, wore male clothing and went to be trained by the famous doctor Herophilus. After she had been trained, still pretending to be a man, she specialized in midwifery and became very successful. Eventually, however, her secret was discovered and she was forced to admit that she had been breaking the law. This accusation angered her female patients and they gave her so much support that the Athenians changed the law in about 300 BCE to allow women (but not slaves) to learn the science of medicine.

A visit from the doctor

Greek physicians could find a lot of advice in the Hippocratic Collection on how to behave towards their patients. In *On Behaviour* they were advised:

"You must visit your patients often and must be careful when you examine them. When you enter a patient's room, be calm and remember your bedside manners. Sometimes the patient may need scolding, sometimes comforting."

Doctors were advised to be cheerful, to avoid wearing strong perfumes and expensive clothes, in case this suggested they were more interested in making money than healing the patient. They were also told not to discuss their fees at the bedside.

The doctor's first task was to observe the patient and ask questions about the symptoms. Then he examined the patient, listening to the lungs, for example, to see if there was any infection. As they had no stethoscopes, they shook the patient and listened to the sounds from inside the body. One book noted that in cases of lung disease a sound 'like leather' could be heard from the lungs.

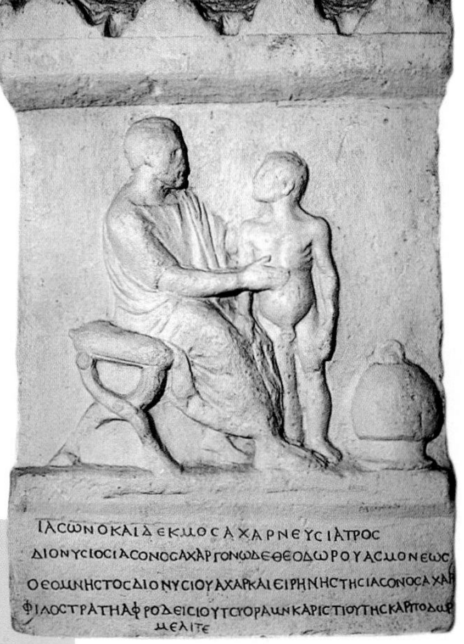

An Athenian physician examining a patient by pressing gently on his stomach.

Examining the patient

First of all the doctor should look at the patient's face. If he looks his usual self, this is a good sign. If not, however, the following are bad signs – a sharp (pointed) nose, hollow eyes, dry skin on the forehead, strange face colour such as green, black, red or lead-coloured. If the face is like this at the beginning of the illness, the doctor must ask the patient if he has lost sleep or had diarrhoea, or not eaten.

From *On Forecasting Diseases*, Section 2

Keeping records and forecasting

Once the doctor had examined the patient, he made detailed notes of the symptoms. This led to the most important part of the doctor's work, forecasting how the illness would develop. This forecast was based on the doctor's experience and his records of similar cases. The evidence shows that Greek doctors took great care to keep detailed records, even when the patient could not be cured. You can read below one doctor's set of case-notes taken from *On Epidemics*, one of the titles in the Hippocratic Collection.

The case-notes of a Greek doctor

At Larisa, a bald man suddenly had a pain in the right thigh. Of the treatments, none helped.
Day 1: sharp burning fever, he did not tremble, but the pains persisted.
Day 2: the pains in the thigh abated, but the fever was worse. He became restless and did not sleep; his extremities were cold. He passed a lot of urine but this was not of the favourable kind.
Day 3: the pain in the thigh stopped. His mind was deranged, with disturbance and much tossing about.
Day 4: near midday, he died.

Exercise and keeping clean

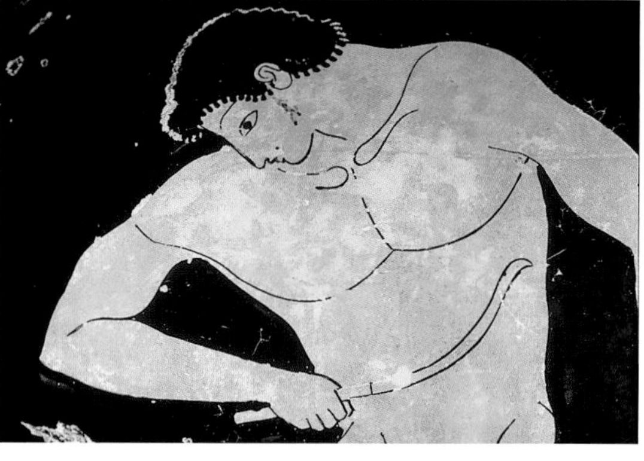

This Greek vase painting depicts a young Athenian athlete using a *strigil* to clean himself.

The most famous evidence for the Greeks' enjoyment of exercise comes from the history of the Olympic Games. The first games were held at Olympia in 776 BCE in honour of Zeus. Stadia were built all over Greece, where athletes won glory for themselves and their cities by competing in wrestling, throwing events and races.

Greek doctors believed that exercise was vital for good health and could cure health problems. Patients were given lengthy advice about how to take care of themselves. This advice is from Diocles of Carystus, a doctor who lived in Athens at the end of the fourth century BCE.

"After awakening he should not arise at once but should wait until the heaviness of sleep has gone. After arising he should rub the whole body with some oil. Thereafter he should every day, wash face and eyes with the hands using pure water. He should rub his teeth inside and outside with the fingers using some fine peppermint powder and cleaning the teeth of remnants of food. He should anoint nose and ears inside, preferably with well-perfumed oil. He should rub and anoint his head every day but wash it and comb it only at intervals. After such a morning toilet, people who are obliged to work will do so but people of leisure will first take a walk. The cultivation of health begins with the moment a man wakes up. A young or middle-aged man should take a walk of about 10 stadia just before sunrise. Long walks before meals clear out the body, prepare it for receiving food and give it more power for digesting."

A young Athenian athlete prepares to throw the discus. Sports like these were part of the school day for all Athenian boys aged 6 to 14, including running, jumping, javelin throwing and wrestling.

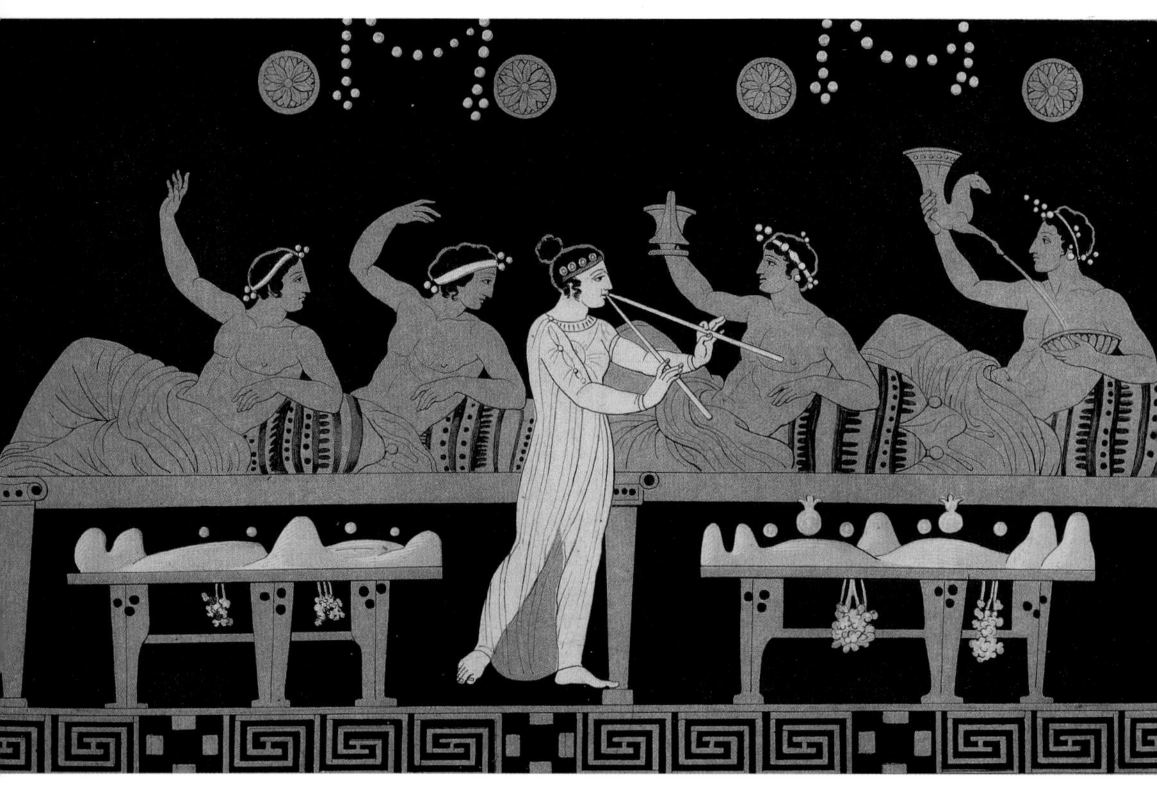

A decorative illustration on a Greek vase shows diners being entertained by a flute player at a banquet. The diners appear to be ignoring the advice of Hippocrates on not eating or drinking too much!

Advice on diet

Doctors also believed that a balanced diet was vital for staying healthy. *A Programme for Health*, another book in the Hippocratic Collection, advised:

"A wise man should consider that health is the greatest of human blessings. In winter, people should eat as much as possible and drink as little as possible – unwatered wine, bread, roast meat and few vegetables. This will keep the body hot and dry. In summer they should drink more and eat less – watered wine, barley cakes and boiled meat so that the body will stay cold and moist. Walking should be fast in winter and slow in summer."

Treatments and cures

What happened if exercise and diet did not cure the patient? Only then did the doctor use other remedies. Greek doctors believed that 'nature itself is the best healer', so they were unwilling to use more drastic methods unless they were clearly necessary. Herbal remedies were an important part of the doctor's armoury of cures. In *On Behaviour,* doctors were told: "A doctor must be able to remember all the drugs and their uses. You must prepare your medicine in good time."

Bleeding and purging

The doctor's aim was always to restore the balance of the patient's humours. If this could not be done by more natural methods, then the doctor would try to remove the excess humour by bleeding the patient, purging his bowels or trying to make him vomit. Doctors bled patients by using a bleeding cup. The warm cup was placed over a small cut and, as the cup cooled, it caused blood to flow out which filled the cup.

Did herbal remedies work?

The story about visiting the *Asclepion* that you read on page 11 also contains an example of using plants as cures. The story tells how the god Asclepios ...

... mixed an ointment for Neoclides, a blind man, by crushing together garlic, verjuice and squills and adding vinegar. This ointment he placed on the man's eyes.

If the man's 'blindness' was caused by an infection that caused his eyes to close up, then this treatment might well have helped. We now know that garlic acts like an antibiotic killing infections, while vinegar cleans wounds like an antiseptic. 'Verjuice' is the juice of unripe fruit such as green apples and a 'squill' is a plant used in a wide range of cures.

A bleeding cup found in a set of Greek medical instruments. Bleeding was such a common treatment that cups were often used as a symbol in illustrations to show that a person was a doctor as, for example, in the picture on page 37.

Was surgery successful?

Physicians who were followers of Hippocrates left surgery to their inferiors, the surgeons – a separate group of doctors. The word 'surgeon' comes from the Latin word *chirurgia*, which itself was based on two Greek words *cheiros* meaning 'craft' and *ergon* meaning 'work'. Surgery was therefore 'craftwork' and regarded as inferior to the brainwork required by physicians, who recorded symptoms and forecasted the development of an illness.

Surgeons did, however, develop good practical methods for dealing with injuries. They set broken bones effectively and could put dislocated joints back into place. They washed wounds with wine or vinegar, which acted like antiseptics and reduced the chances of infection. Sometimes they also bandaged wounds with linen soaked in wine.

Surgery inside the body was the last resort, when the physician's attempts to restore the

This fresco from the city of Pompeii shows a surgeon dealing with a wound during the Trojan War.

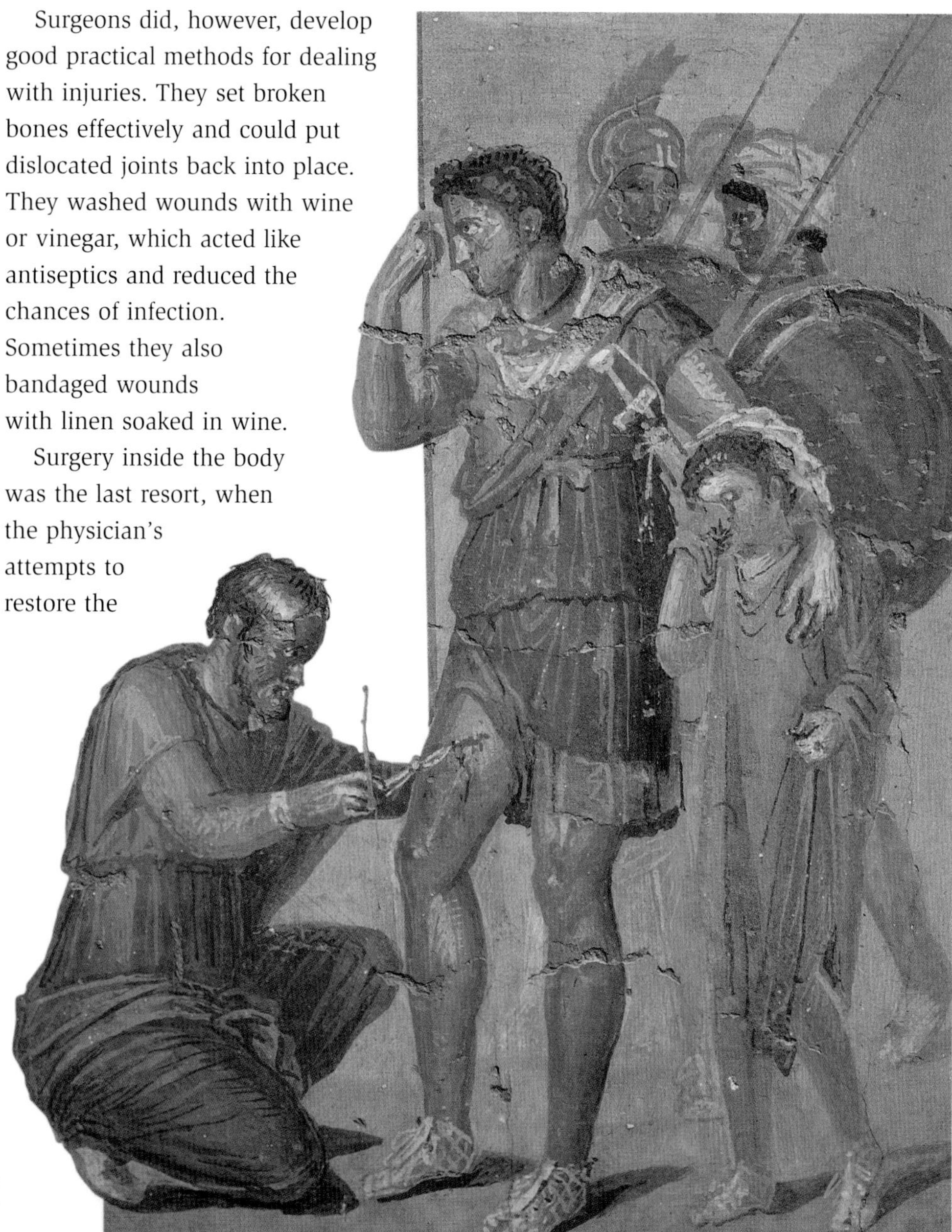

balance of the patient's humours had failed. Surgeons knew that there was a great deal they did not understand about the body. They could not stop heavy bleeding and they had no effective anaesthetics, although wine and drugs such as hemlock may have been used to dull pain.

The books in the Hippocratic Collection do, however, show a good deal of knowledge about surgery. Surgeons are advised about where to position the patient and their instruments so that they could work in a good light. One common internal operation was the draining of the lungs of patients with pneumonia. This operation was carefully described in medical books and successfully carried out many times. Doctors also performed more dangerous surgery in emergencies. There is evidence that the Greeks amputated limbs when they could see that a limb was rotten with gangrene. There are also detailed descriptions in Hippocratic texts of how to undertake a procedure known as 'trepanning'. When a patient had sustained a serious head injury, the surgeon needed to relieve the pressure on the brain by cutting or drilling into the skull.

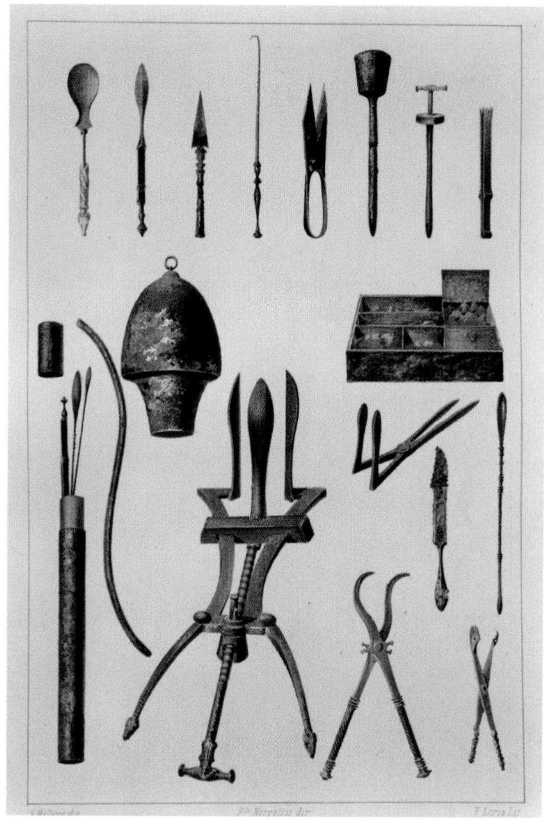

Greek surgical instruments were stronger and sharper than earlier surgical instruments, thanks to the development of iron and steel-making *c.* 1200 BCE.

Wounds and surgery in *The Iliad*

Homer's epic poem *The Iliad* gives us the first evidence of battle wounds in history. The story of the attack on Troy is full of battle scenes and Homer describes 147 battle wounds. Of these, 106 were sword thrusts, 17 were sword slashes, 12 were arrow shots and there were 12 slingshots. The great majority of the wounded died, but one survivor was King Menelaus. He was hit in the waist by an arrow, but the doctor drew out the arrow, cleaned the wound and applied a healing ointment.

Chapter 5

From the Greeks to the Romans

The key ideas of Greek medicine

Some Greek medical methods were similar to methods used by the Egyptians and other early peoples. Women dealt with most of the medical problems at home. Herbal remedies were widely used, both in the home and by physicians, and many of them would have been effective, having been tried and tested over many years. Religion also played a large part in Greek medicine. Many people travelled long distances to be treated at the temples of the god of medicine, Asclepios, where the priests provided a wide range of treatments.

Greek medicine was not, however, identical to medicine in earlier societies. Following the ideas of the legendary figure of Hippocrates, physicians developed their theories and wrote down their observations and treatments. The Hippocratic Collection of medical books had a

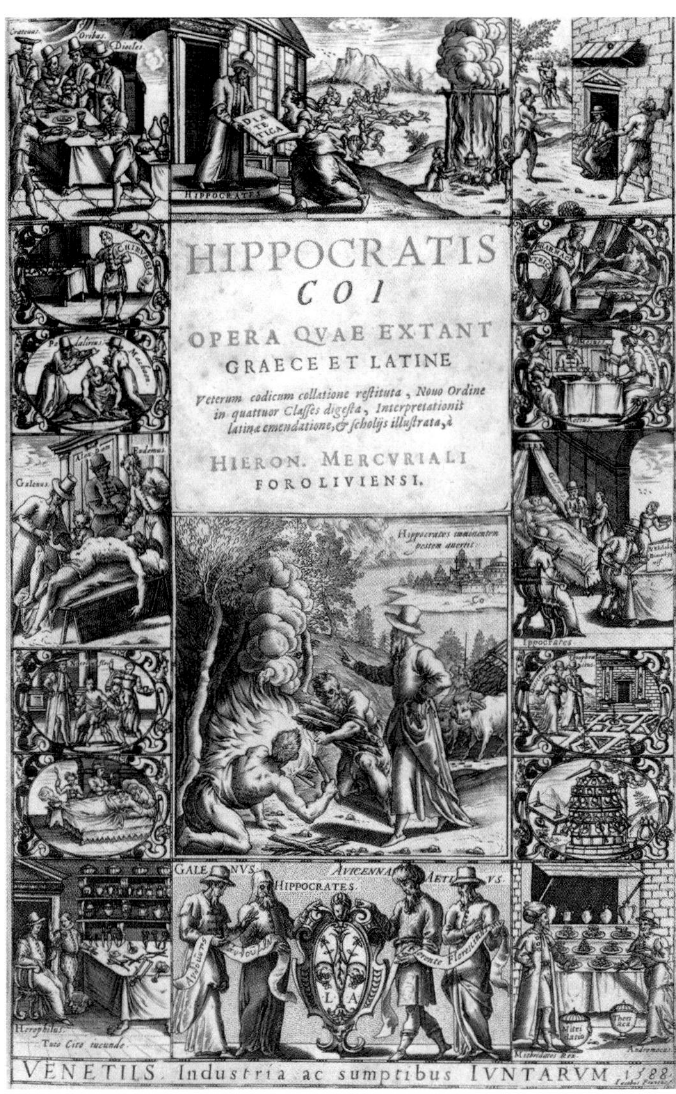

HIPPOCRATIS COI

OPERA QVAE EXTANT GRAECE ET LATINE

Veterum codicum collatione restituta, Nouo Ordine in quattuor Classes digesta, Interpretationis latinae emendatione, & scholijs illustrata, à

HIERON. MERCVRIALI FOROLIVIENSI.

VENETIIS. Industria ac sumptibus IVNTARVM, 1588.

This edition of the works of Hippocrates was published in Venice in 1588. The medical ideas of the Greeks were still accepted as correct two thousand years after Hippocrates lived.

huge influence on later doctors. Above all, Greek doctors were practical. They advised their patients on how to avoid illness, recommending rest, exercise and a good diet. If a patient fell ill, the doctor carefully observed the pattern of the illness, recorded the symptoms and compared them to the case-histories of other patients.

Greek doctors did not abandon their belief that the gods had some role in illness, but they believed that there were natural, rational reasons for illness. People became sick when the body's humours were out of balance. Therefore the doctor's role was to restore the proper balance of the patients' humours and so make them well again.

Greek medical ideas and treatments continued to be accepted as correct for centuries, partly due to the work of Claudius Galen, a Roman who built on and developed the work of Hippocrates and other Greek physicians.

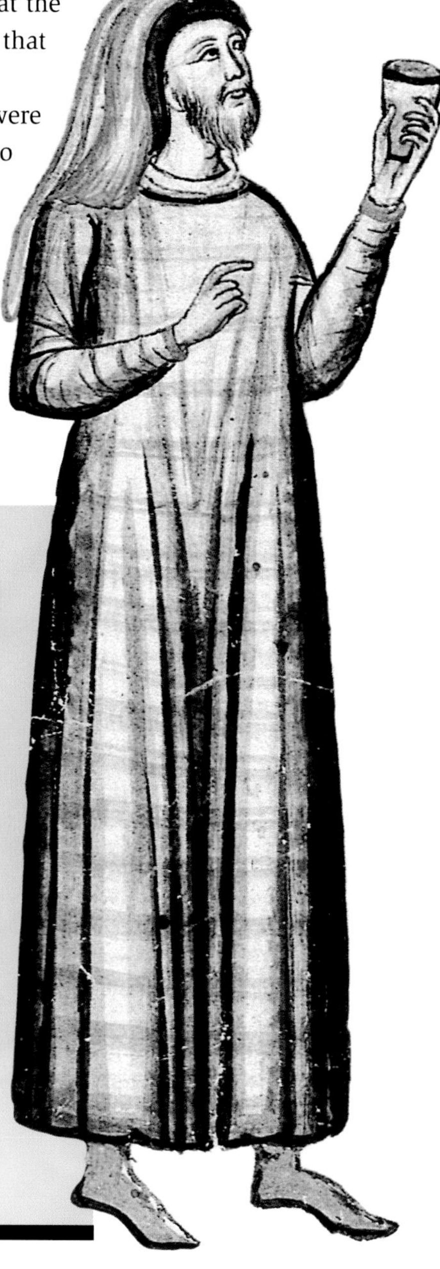

A medieval Arabic illustration of Hippocrates inspecting a urine jar. Hippocrates' works were well known among Arab scholars.

Explanations for epidemics

Greek doctors did not pretend that they could cure every illness, otherwise why did so many people become sick at the same time during an epidemic? Their humours could not all become unbalanced at the same time! In Athens in 430–427 BCE there were numerous different explanations for the sudden outbreak of plague. One suggestion was that the cause must be in the air, because breathing air was the only thing that people had in common. Huge bonfires were lit to 'improve' the air. People also blamed the gods for the plague or said that their enemies, the Spartans, had poisoned the water wells. Another theory, the closest of all, was that overcrowding in the hot city spread the disease. Yet this theory did not explain how the plague began.

The growth of the Roman Empire

The Roman Empire became the most powerful empire in the ancient world. Around 750 BCE the Romans were simply the people who lived in villages overlooking the River Tiber. These villages gradually grew into the city of Rome and by 250 BCE Rome's soldiers had conquered the whole of Italy. Five hundred years later, they ruled most of Europe, including Greece, North Africa and large parts of the Middle East.

Rome's success was due to its huge, efficient army. It had by far the best-trained, best-equipped and most disciplined soldiers. With their short, stabbing swords, they fought in well-organized formations and were too powerful for the wild, brave but usually unplanned attacks of their opponents. Rebels, such as Boudicca in Britain, were briefly successful, but they could not match the strength and resources of the Roman army for long.

The Romans also built an extensive road network, which helped their army move swiftly to trouble spots and speeded up trade. Most people in the Empire soon

This map highlights the extent of the Roman Empire at its peak *c.* 120–250 CE.

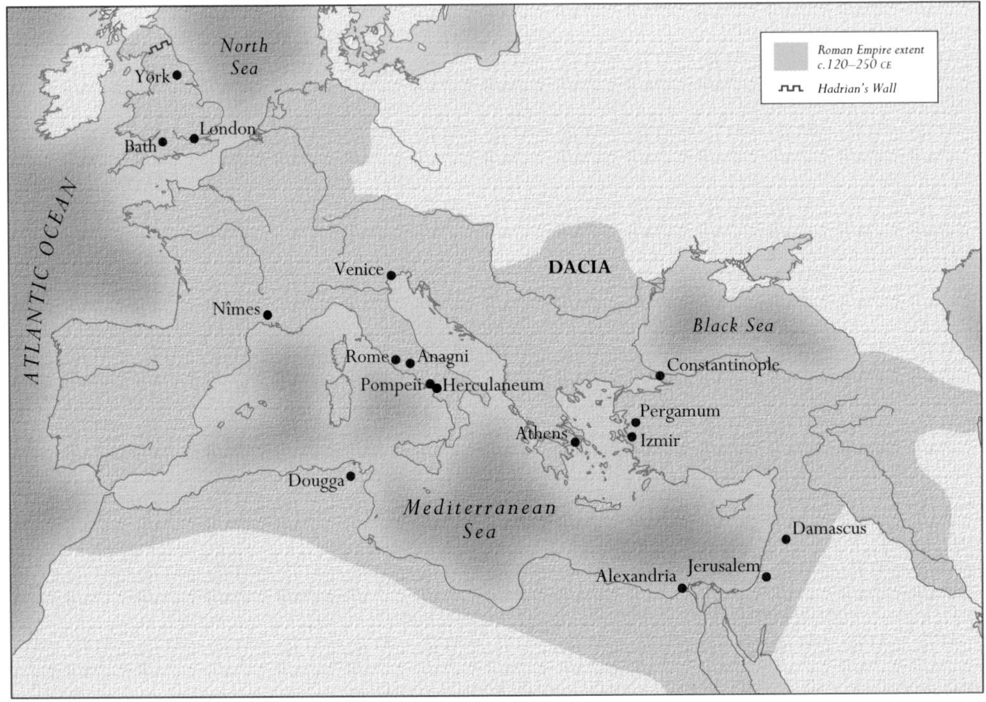

The practical Romans

What were the differences between the Greeks and the Romans? One vital difference was the Roman interest in engineering. The Greeks had studied geometry and mathematics for their own sakes, but the Romans put them to good use in engineering. Strabo, the Greek geographer, summed up the difference between the two peoples:

The Greeks are famous for their cities and they aimed at beauty. The Romans excelled in those things in which the Greeks took little interest, such as the building of roads, aqueducts and sewers.

enjoyed the advantages of being connected to Rome. They could buy a wider range of better-quality goods, thanks to stronger trading links. Towns, such as London and Lyons, developed – a sure sign of prosperity and flourishing trade. Local leaders copied the customs and living standards of Rome by learning Latin and going to amphitheatres to watch gladiatorial shows. And, by allowing local peoples to keep their own gods and goddesses, the Romans reduced the likelihood of rebellions.

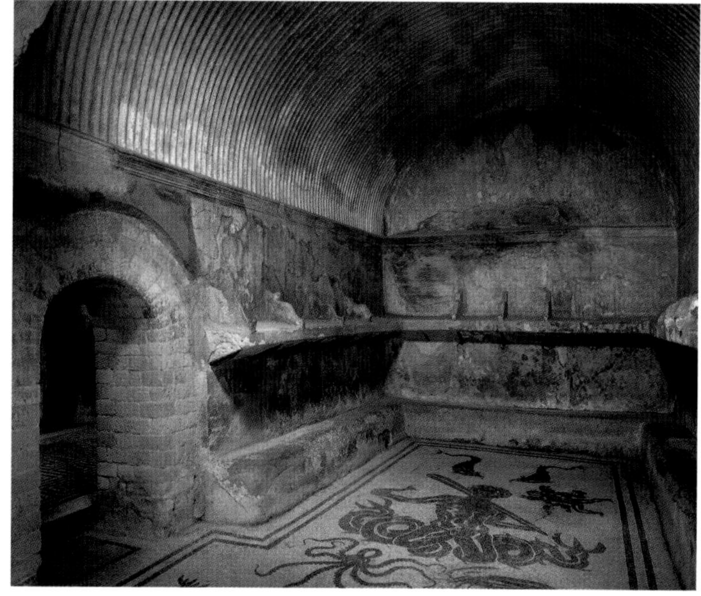

The women's hall in the baths at Herculaneum in Italy. The solidity of the stonework and the decorative mosaic demonstrate the quality of Roman building skills.

These aspects of the Roman world all had an effect on their medical ideas and treatments. The Romans were very inventive and practical people. Great efforts were put into keeping their army healthy because, without it, the Roman Empire would crumble. Their engineering and building skills were used to pipe fresh water and build sewers – both vital parts of public health schemes. Trade and war brought ideas from other countries, including Greece, which was the homeland of many of the first doctors in the city of Rome.

Chapter 6

How did the Romans try to heal the sick?

The Roman gods of healing

In 295 BCE the people of Rome were struck down by a severe plague. Household remedies failed to stop the plague spreading and appeals to the Roman goddess of health, Salus, did not have any effect. In desperation, the Romans turned to Asclepios, the Greek god of healing. They built a temple to the god and imported a sacred snake from Greece – and then the plague faded away. So Asclepios became an accepted part of healing in the Roman Empire. Romans started to pray and make sacrifices to Asclepios as well as Salus, asking for good health and for cures.

A Roman altar dedicated to Asclepios and to the Roman goddess of health, Salus. This altar was found in Britain and dates from the second century CE.

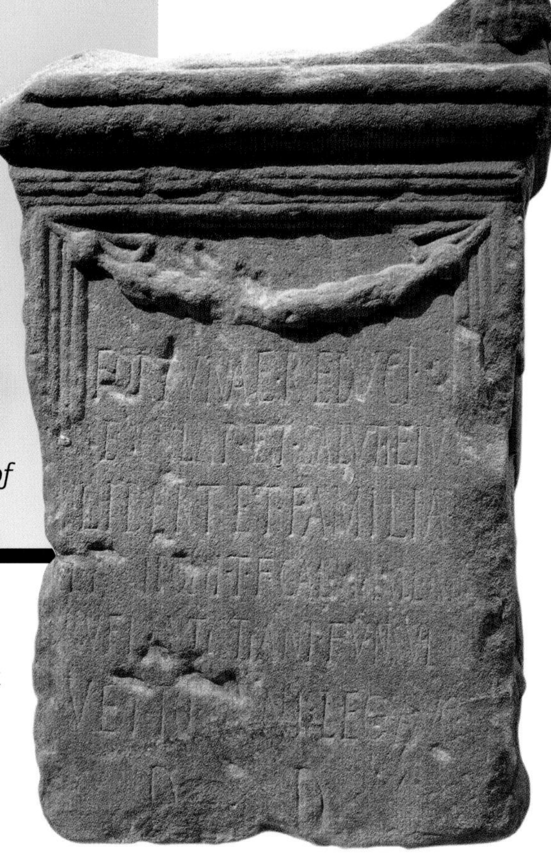

Roman gods of healing

Here are some inscriptions on Roman altars found in Britain. Prayers to the gods were the only form of health insurance available!

To the holy god Asclepios and to Hygeia, Julius Saturninus set this [altar] up.

To the mighty saviour gods, I, Hermogenes, a doctor, set up this altar.

To Asclepios and Salus for the welfare of the cavalry regiment.

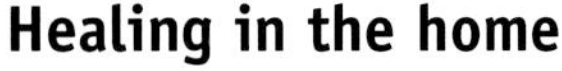

Healing in the home

Like the Greeks, the Romans expected that most medical care would be given in the home. They prayed to their household gods for good health and cures, but they also believed that the *pater familias*, the head of the household, knew enough about herbal remedies and other practical remedies to take care of his family and slaves. Of course, the women of the household played a major part in this everyday medicine too. Pliny the Elder, a Roman who wrote a huge encyclopaedia about science and nature *c.* 75 CE, paid women a back-handed compliment when he said: "The science of charms and herbs is the one outstanding skill of women".

Wealthy Romans owned medical books to advise them on treatments. One popular medical encyclopaedia was *Artes*, 'The Sciences', by Celsus. He was a wealthy landowner who built up his knowledge partly by treating his own family and friends. Celsus provided guidance on everything from diet to surgery and on symptoms and treatments affecting every part of the body from the head to the toes. Like many other writers, both Greek and Roman, he stressed the importance of exercise as a way of avoiding illness:

"He who has been busy during the day, whether in domestic or public affairs, ought to put aside some part of the day for the care of the body. The most important way to care for the body is through exercise, which ought to come to an end with sweating."

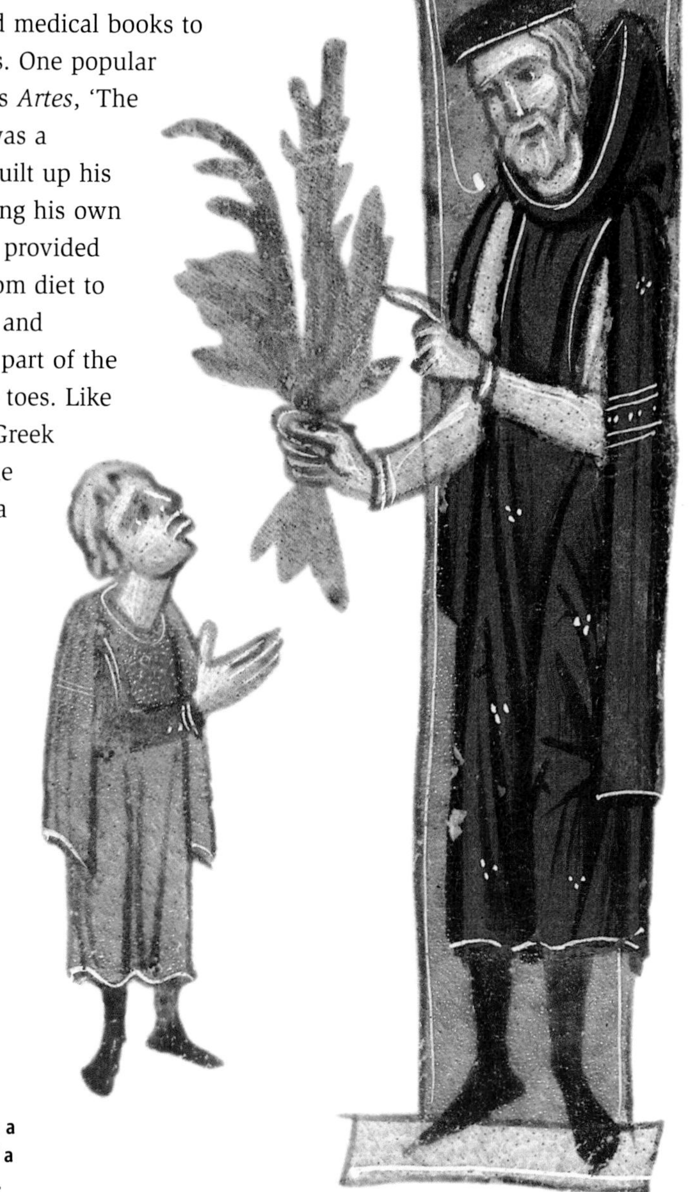

The same herbal remedies were used for many centuries. This medieval illustration comes from a thirteenth-century translation of a book by the Roman doctor Galen.

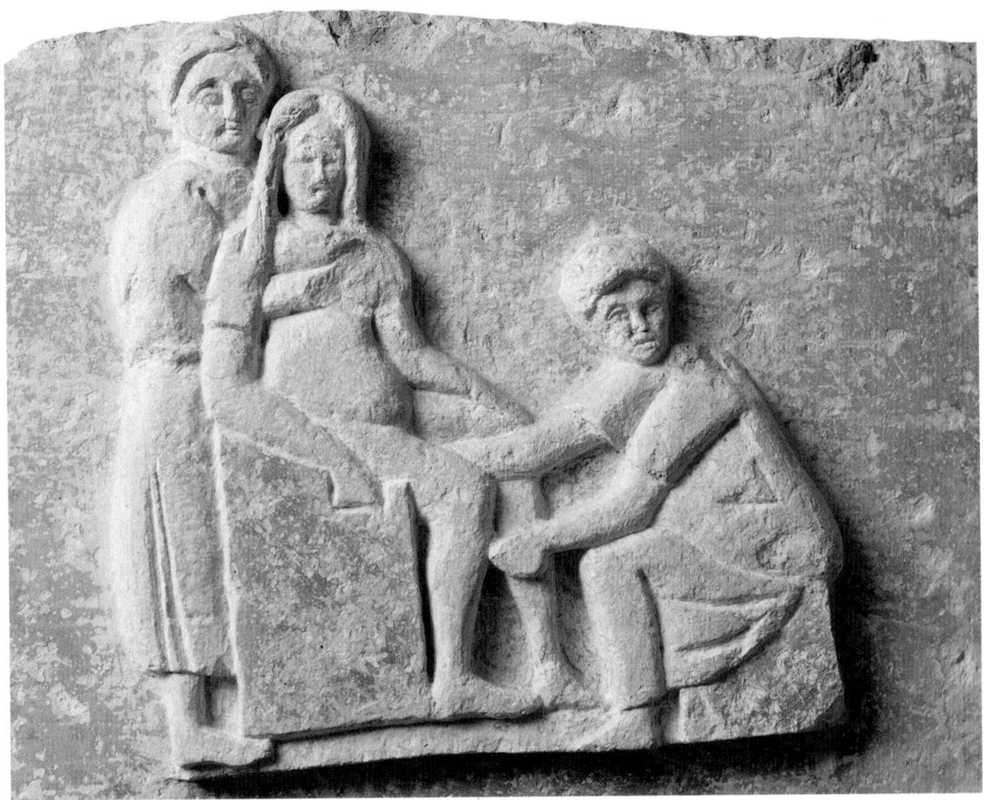

This second-century carving shows a midwife and her assistant delivering a baby. While many midwives had plenty of experience, they had no technical methods of helping if there were problems during a birth. One piece of advice was for four people to take hold of the mother and shake her violently ten times to speed the birth.

Herbal treatments

The Roman father, as head of the household, could look up herbal treatments in a huge compendium compiled by Dioscorides around 64 CE. Dioscorides was a Greek surgeon in Emperor Nero's army. Modern scientific tests have shown that at least twenty per cent of the remedies in the compendium contained ingredients like honey and garlic that helped patients, because they killed the bacteria in infections.

Women doctors and midwives

By the first century BCE, many cities employed doctors to treat the poor. Some of these doctors were women. One, Antiochus, was so successful that a statue was erected in her hometown in "recognition of her skill as a medical practitioner". Women also continued to act as midwives. According to the medical writer Soranus, the best midwives were intelligent, robust, respectable and literate and experienced in nutrition, pharmacy and surgery. Handbooks on midwifery emphasized the importance of cleanliness, listing the need for sponges, wool coverings, bandages, and oil and hot water for cleansing. This advice would have been far more use than that from Pliny the Elder, who advocated reducing labour pains by hurling a projectile, preferably a cavalry spear, three times over the roof of the house!

A Roman doctor inspecting the eye of a patient. This carving also shows two bleeding cups.

Surgery

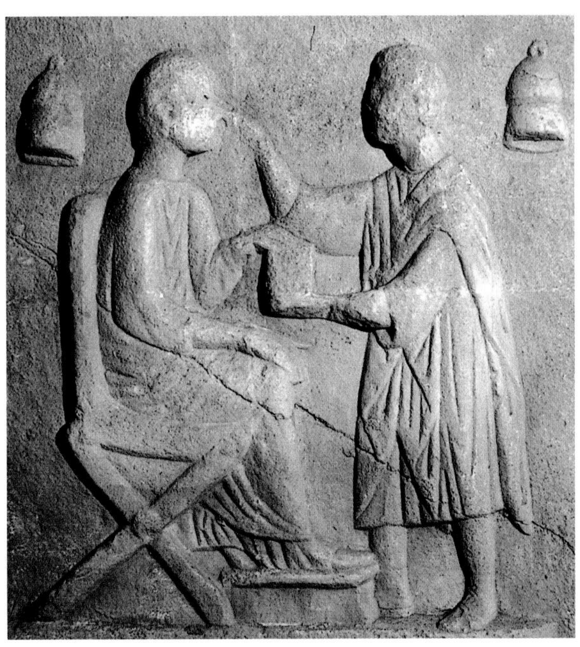

Surgical skills and methods were still very much based on military experience. Each legion had its own doctor and medical orderlies, who learned how to deal with all levels of wounds from simple cuts to spear and arrow wounds, dislocations and even amputations. Internal operations were rare, but some surgeons did develop specialist skills, such as removing cataracts from eyes with exceptionally fine needles. In this case the gravest danger was the patient moving.

Pliny's remedies

Here are some remedies from Pliny the Elder's book, *Natural History*:

- *Unwashed wool, applied with honey, heals old sores and heals wounds if dipped in wine and vinegar. Yolks of eggs can be taken for dysentery, mixed with poppy juice and wine.*
- *The saliva of a fasting human being is the best of all safeguards against snakes, but our daily experience may teach us even more valuable ways of using it. We spit on epileptics having a fit, because that is throwing back the infection. In a similar way we ward off witchcraft and the bad luck that follows meeting someone who is lame in the right leg.*

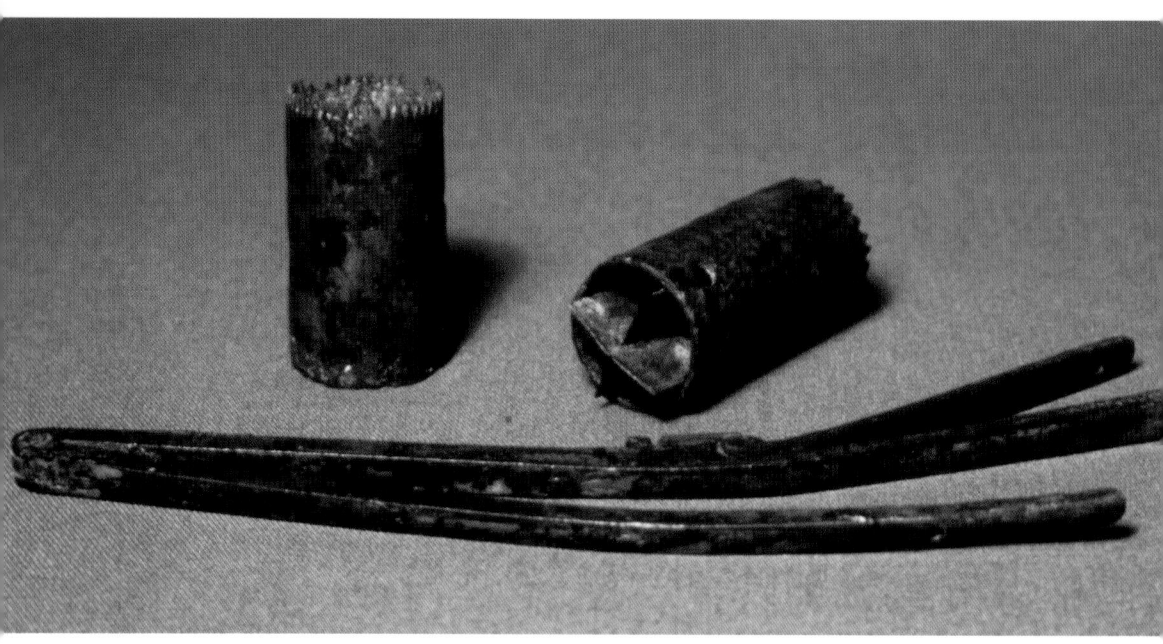

Trepanning equipment found in Britain. Trepanning involves cutting a hole in the skull using saw-edged tools such as the ones shown here. The method had been used previously by prehistoric peoples who used flint knives. Skulls found in Britain from the Roman period show that healing took place after the operation. Very similar instruments were still used in the nineteenth century.

Amputations and anaesthetics

On rare occasions, surgeons did amputate limbs when everything else had failed. Celsus described one operation like this:

"When gangrene has developed, the limb must be amputated. But even that involves very great risk, for patients often die under the operation. It does not matter, however, whether the remedy is safe because it is the only one. Therefore the flesh is cut through with a scalpel down to the bone, between the sound and the diseased parts. This must not be done over a joint and it is better that some of the sound flesh should be cut away than that any of the diseased part be left behind. The bone is then cut through with a small saw ..."

Surgeons tried to anaesthetize their patients with herbal drugs such as henbane or mandrake to reduce pain and to make the operations easier to carry out. Celsus provided a recipe that said:

"Take a good handful of wild poppy-heads when just ripe for collecting the juice and put into a vessel and boil

with sufficient water to cover it. When this handful has been well boiled, squeeze it out and throw it away. Take the juice and mix it with an equal quantity of raisin wine and heat the mixture. When the mixture has cooled, pills are formed. These will make the patient sleep."

The pills had some effect, although there was always the danger of giving the patient so many that they never woke up!

Another major danger during surgery was infection. This could actually have been a greater danger for the patients of wealthy surgeons, as their medical instruments were specially made with inlaid patterns in the metal. The patterns simply attracted and held germs (which the Romans were unaware of), whereas poorer surgeons had the simplest and, therefore, potentially the cleanest instruments.

A Roman surgeon's knife made from bronze and iron. Roman surgical instruments were well-designed for the simple surgery carried out. Surgeons in the twentieth century had no difficulty identifying what each instrument was used for because their own instruments were very similar.

The qualities of a surgeon

A surgeon should be youthful or at any rate nearer youth than age; with a strong and steady hand which never trembles, and ready to use the left hand as well as the right; with vision sharp and clear, and spirit undaunted; filled with pity; so that he wishes to cure the patient, yet is not moved by his cries, to go too fast, or cut less than is necessary; but he does everything just as if the cries of pain cause him no emotion.

Celsus, *De Medicina*, Book VII

Chapter 7

Why was Galen so important?

Greek doctors in Rome

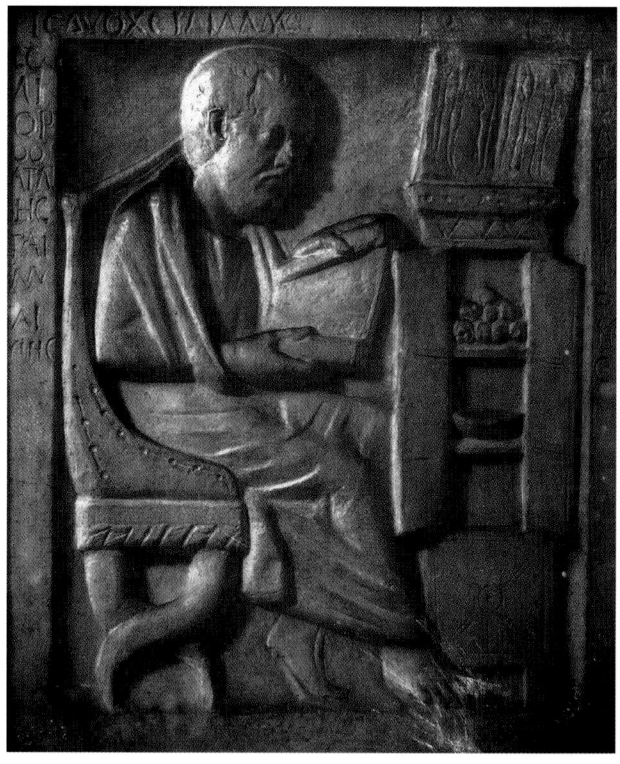

A Greek doctor consults his scrolls, which give details of his patients' records.

The first Greek doctors arrived in Rome by 200 BCE. They were prisoners of war who had been captured when the Roman army conquered the Greek Empire. They were then bought by wealthy Romans to treat their families and slaves. By the first century BCE, many were freed and so they set themselves up in business as doctors in Rome. As Rome grew more prosperous, other Greek doctors arrived, hoping to make their fortunes.

It soon became the fashion for wealthy Romans to have Greek doctors. Roman doctors even took Greek names to get more clients, but some Romans sneered at this new fashion. "Medicine," mocked Pliny the Elder, "changes every day and we are swept along on the puffs of the clever brains of the Greeks. As if thousands of people did not live without physicians – though not, of course, without medicine."

Claudius Galen

Despite the sneers, Roman Emperors employed Greek doctors, including the most famous doctor in Roman history, Claudius Galen. Galen was born in Pergamum in Greece in 131 CE and was the son of a wealthy architect. Galen's father had a dream that his son would become a physician and spent a great deal of money giving Galen the best possible medical education. He even sent him to study at the great medical school in Alexandria. When Galen was eighteen, he became the surgeon at a gladiators' school, which gave him practical experience of dealing with wounds and increased his knowledge of anatomy, as wounds provided "a window into the body".

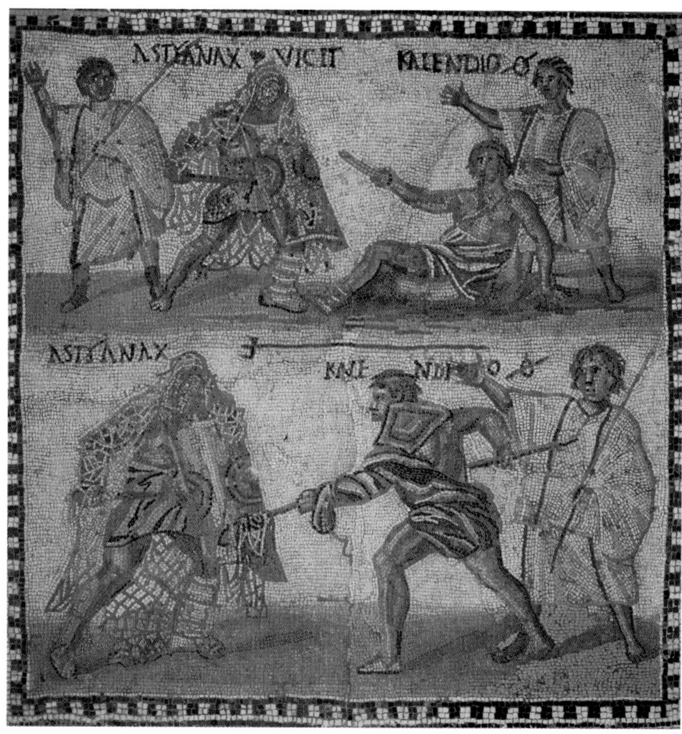

This Roman mosaic from the fourth century CE shows gladiators in action. The most common wounds the gladiators sustained were cuts and broken or dislocated limbs.

Doctor to the Emperor

At the age of twenty, Galen moved to Rome, and quickly became well known, but he also made enemies by mocking and criticizing others. Galen may have inherited his temper from his mother who, he wrote, "used to bite her maids and was always shouting at my father". Older doctors resented his arrogance, forcing him to leave Rome, but he was soon back in the city. When plague broke out, the Emperor Marcus Aurelius summoned Galen to take care of the royal family and protected him from the jealousy of other doctors.

Death by medicine!

This is what the Roman writer Pliny had to say about Greek physicians in Rome:

There is no doubt that all these physicians hunt for popularity by trying new ideas and do not hesitate to buy that popularity with our lives. Hence those wretched quarrelsome consultations at the bedside of the patients. Hence too that gloomy inscription on gravestones, "It was the crowd of physicians which killed me." Only a physician can commit homicide with complete immunity.

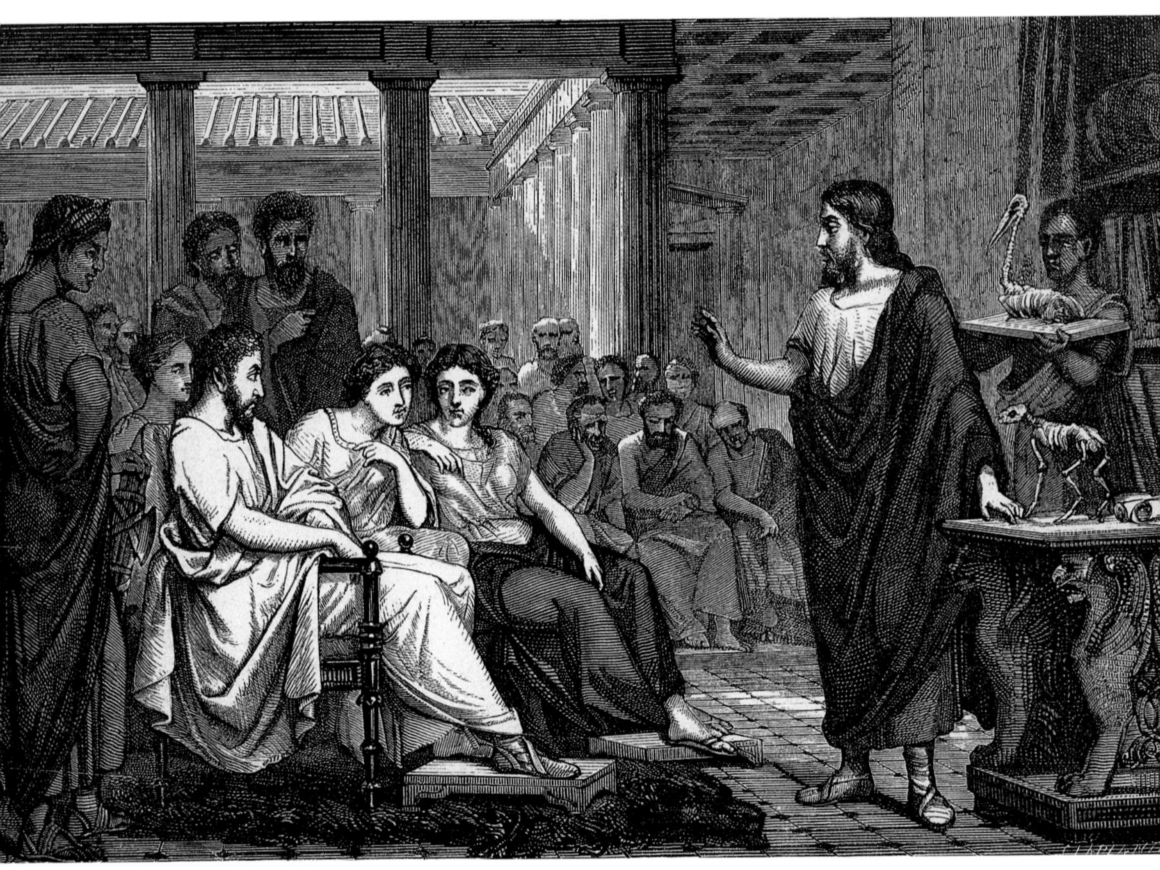

This nineteenth-century engraving recreates a scene showing Galen giving a lecture in Rome using the skeletons of animals as his examples. Illustrations like this and the one on the opposite page show how long-lasting the interest in Galen's work was.

Galen's work

Galen's work was built on the key ideas in the Hippocratic Collection. He emphasized the importance of clinical observation – careful examination of patients and taking detailed notes of their symptoms. He also believed that illness was caused by imbalances in the Four Humours in the body. However, Galen did not just accept the ideas of Hippocrates. He added his own theories and developments.

Galen developed the 'treatment of opposites', a system of treatment that he based on the theory of the Four Humours. He said that if an illness was caused by cold then the patients needed treatments that would heat them up, so he used ingredients such as peppers in his cures. If a disease was caused by heat, then the patient would need a cooling cure, perhaps using cucumber in the medicine or diet.

Opportunities for learning anatomy

If you cannot get to Alexandria, it is not impossible to see human bones. I have often had the chance to do this where tombs have been broken. On one occasion a river caused a grave to disintegrate and then carried the corpse away downstream before depositing it on the riverbank. Here it lay, ready for inspection, just as though prepared by a doctor for his pupils' lesson. Once I also examined the skeleton of a robber lying on a mountainside.

From Galen's *On Anatomy* 190 CE

Galen also believed that physicians should try to find out as much as possible about the structure and workings of the body. He wrote:

"Human bones are the subjects that you should first get to know. You cannot merely read about bones in books, but you must also acquaint yourself with the appearance of each of the bones, by the use of your own eye, handling each bone by itself."

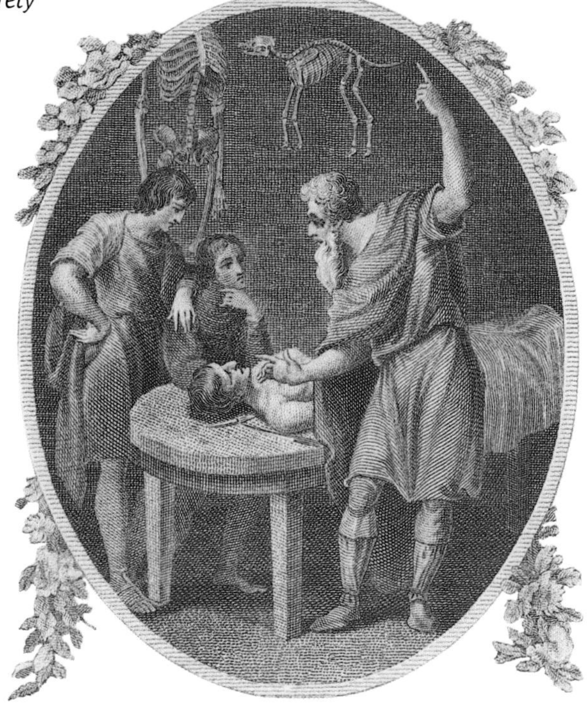

An engraving from 1796 entitled "Galen and patient".

He advised doctors to travel to Alexandria where physicians allowed students to inspect human bodies for themselves even though dissection of human bodies was, in theory, illegal. If this was not possible, he advised doctors to dissect apes:

"For this you should choose apes which most resemble men. These are apes which do not have prominent jaws or large canine teeth. In these apes, which also walk and run on two legs, you will also find the other parts as in man."

Galen the showman

Galen was a showman as well as a scientist. When he arrived in Rome he conducted public dissections of animals in order to win publicity. He knew just how to arrange these dissections to surprise and win over his audiences. One famous experiment was the dissection of a pig to demonstrate the workings of the nervous system. As the pig squirmed and squealed on the table, Galen cut into its neck, finding the nerves. He could have cut through the right nerve immediately to stop the pig squealing, but that did not appeal to Galen's showmanship.

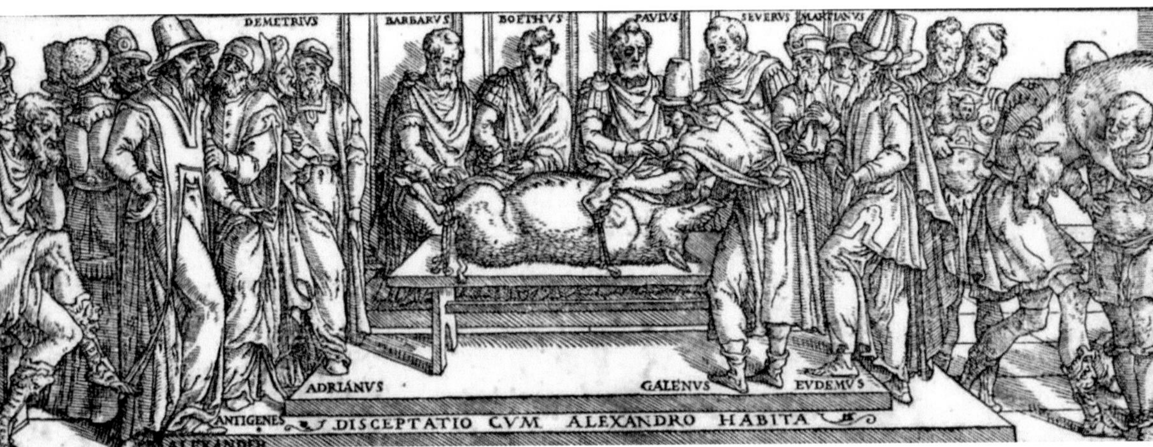

In this medieval illustration, Galen dissects a pig to show the workings of the nervous system.

Instead he announced, "I will cut this nerve but the pig will keep squealing." He cut, and the pig did keep squealing. He cut again, building up the audience's interest and again the pig kept squealing. Then he announced, "When I cut this nerve, the pig will stop squealing." He cut and the pig fell silent!

Although he usually had to dissect animals, not humans, some of Galen's discoveries were important. He proved that the brain, not the heart, controlled speech and that the arteries, and not just the veins, carried blood around the body. Inevitably he made mistakes because the bodies of apes and pigs are not the same as those of humans, but it was to be well over a thousand years before anyone dared to challenge Galen's findings.

Galen's significance

Galen wrote over 60 books, covering every aspect of medicine in an extremely detailed and well-organized way. He included the work of earlier doctors such as Hippocrates, Herophilus and Erasistratus, but he also added his own work on treatments and on the structure and workings of the body. Galen's books became the basis for medical education for the next fifteen hundred years. One important reason why he was so influential was that his ideas fitted in with the ideas of the Christian church, which controlled education in Europe in the Middle Ages. Galen believed that all parts of the body had been produced by a Creator for a definite purpose, matching the Christian belief that God had created human beings.

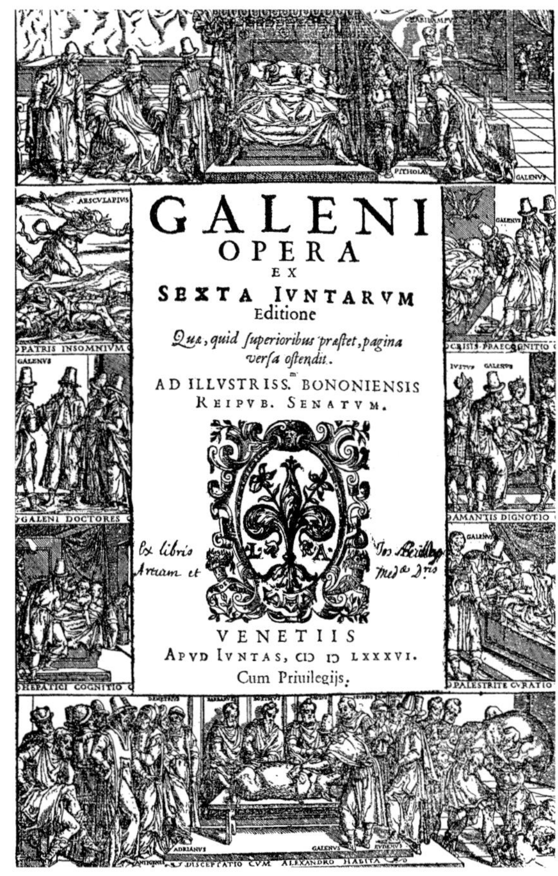

GALENI
OPERA
EX
SEXTA IVNTARVM
Editione
Quae, quid superioribus praestet, pagina versa ostendit.
AD ILLVSTRISS. BONONIENSIS REIPVB. SENATVM.
VENETIIS
APVD IVNTAS, CIϽ IϽ LXXXVI.
Cum Priuilegijs.

The title page of one of Galen's books that was printed and published in Venice in 1586, nearly 1400 years after Galen died.

Galen on Galen

This is Galen's assessment of his own place in medical history. His attitude helps to explain why he was not popular with other doctors. Trajan was Emperor of Rome 98–117 CE and was famous for his military conquests and building projects.

I have done as much for medicine as Trajan did for the Roman Empire when he built bridges and roads through Italy. It is I, and I alone, who have revealed the true path of medicine. It must be admitted that Hippocrates already staked out the path. He prepared the way, but I have made it possible.

Chapter 8

Were the Romans really so clean and healthy?

Why was public health so important?

Roman rulers knew that they needed healthy people to keep the Empire strong. Soldiers obviously had to be fit and healthy, but so too did farm workers and merchants – the people whose work kept the Empire fed and prosperous. Therefore public health schemes – water supplies, baths and sewerage systems – were built

The Roman bath-house at Chesters fort on Hadrian's Wall, Northumberland, built *c.* 125 CE. The site for the fort was carefully chosen as it was near a river, which provided fresh water.

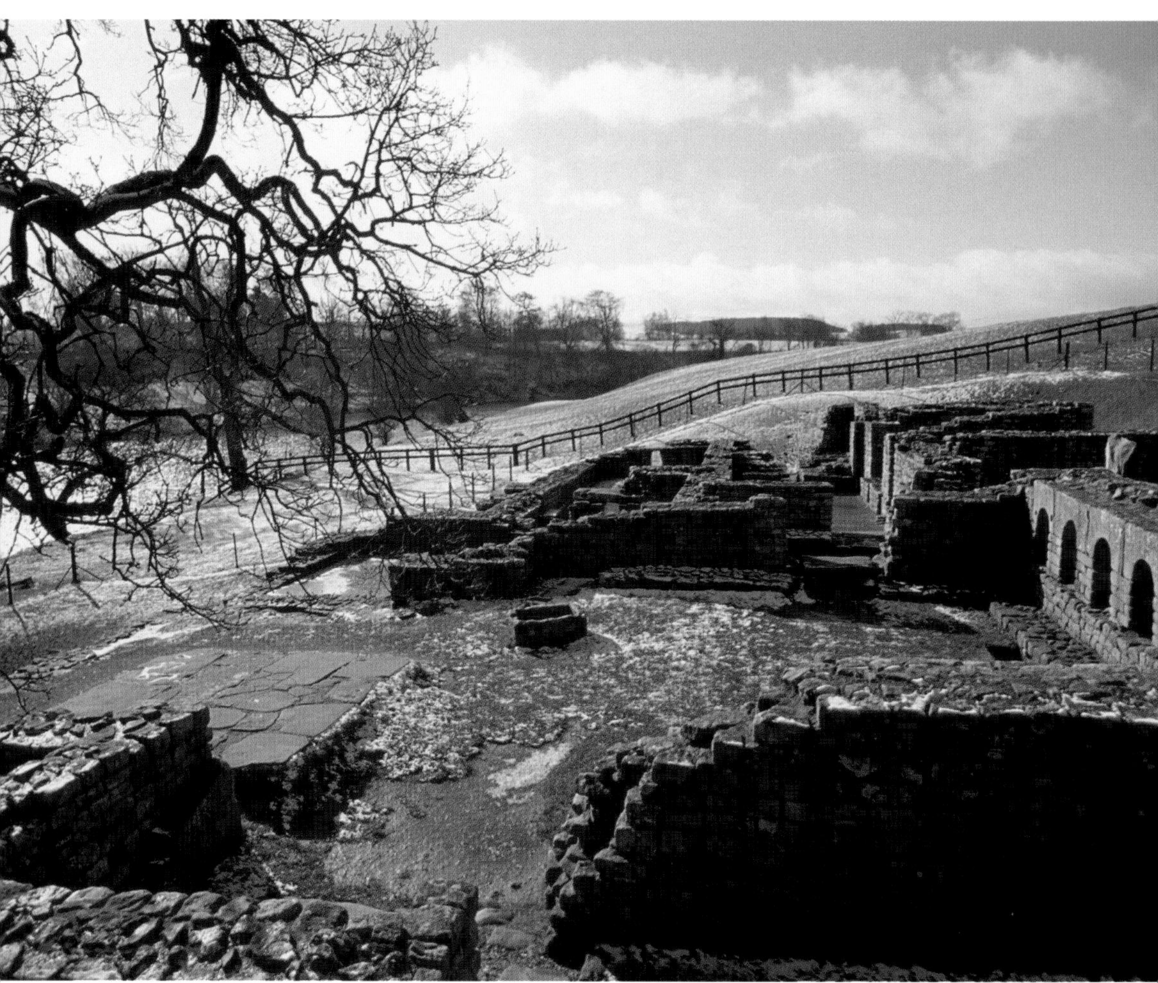

throughout the Empire. Sometimes slaves captured in war were used as the labour force. On other occasions, a local workforce was employed, paid out of the taxes the Romans collected so efficiently. Once buildings were in use, engineers, often from the army, kept everything running and dealt with repairs. These schemes were a tribute to the high quality of Roman organization.

Siting a military camp

It was particularly important to protect the army from disease. The military writer, Vegetius, gave this advice to army commanders:

Soldiers must not remain too long near unhealthy marshes. A soldier must not drink swamp water. If a group of soldiers is allowed to stay in one place too long in summer or autumn then they begin to suffer from the effects of polluted water and are made miserable by the smell of their own excrement. The air becomes unhealthy and they catch diseases. This has to be put right by moving to another camp.

Healthy sites for towns and forts

The Romans knew that it was important to build their towns, villas or army forts in healthy places. In his book, *Country Life*, Marcus Varro advised:

"When building a house or farm, especial care should be taken to place it at the foot of a wooded hill where it is exposed to health-giving winds. Care should be taken when there are swamps in the neighbourhood, because certain tiny creatures, which cannot be seen by the eyes, breed there. These float through the air and enter the body through the mouth and nose and cause serious diseases."

Another writer, Columella, noted that, in summer, marshlands "give birth to animals with mischief-making stings which fly at us in thick swarms." Clearly, Romans were well aware of the dangers of mosquitoes and malaria.

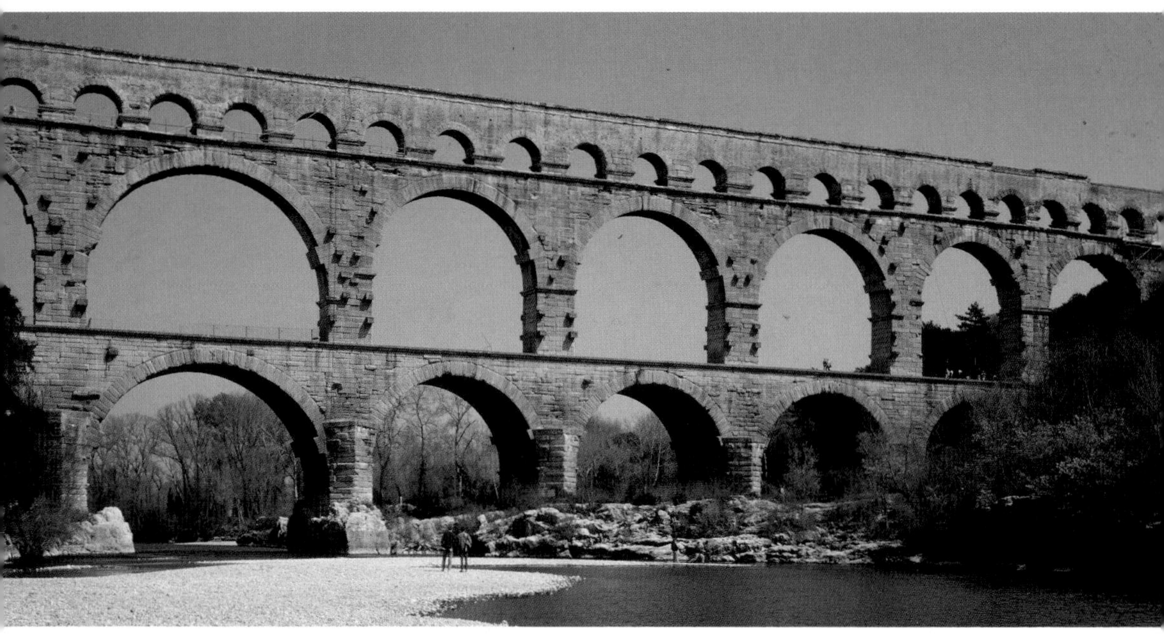

The Roman aqueduct Pont du Gard in Nîmes, France.

Solving the problem of water

The Romans also built their settlements near good, fresh water supplies but, as time went by, towns grew rapidly and more water was needed. This created the problem of how to transport water over long distances. Engineers solved this problem by building brick or stone tunnels called 'conduits' to carry the water long distances. Once the water reached a town reservoir, small bronze or lead pipes could take it short distances to public baths or fountains.

However, this did not solve all the problems. Firstly, the conduits had to be built extremely carefully on a very gentle slope so that the water ran slowly but freely to its destination. Secondly, what happened when the engineers came to a valley? They could not have water in a conduit running steeply down and then uphill! The answer was to build aqueducts, or bridges, which carried the conduits across valleys. In other places, engineers dug out tunnels through hills to keep the water supplies flowing.

These kinds of engineering feats took place right across the Empire. In Britain, for example, aqueducts were often less visually dramatic but were just as effective. Most towns received their water supplies from clay-lined channels that had been dug into the ground. The channel supplying Dorchester in England was nearly 13 kilometres long, 1.5 metres wide and 91 centimetres deep. The aqueduct at Wroxeter in Shropshire delivered 9.1 million litres of water a day. Main pipelines, made of timber and lead, ran along the major streets of the town and then side channels diverted the water into individual buildings. If there was a drought, the supply to individual buildings could be cut off, ensuring that supplies would last as long as possible. Most people also stored water in wells or in barrels outside their houses.

The Romans discovered how to make concrete, which enabled them to build bigger, stronger structures. The Colosseum in Rome was built in 70–83 CE. Here the Romans watched gladiatorial combat and other entertainment.

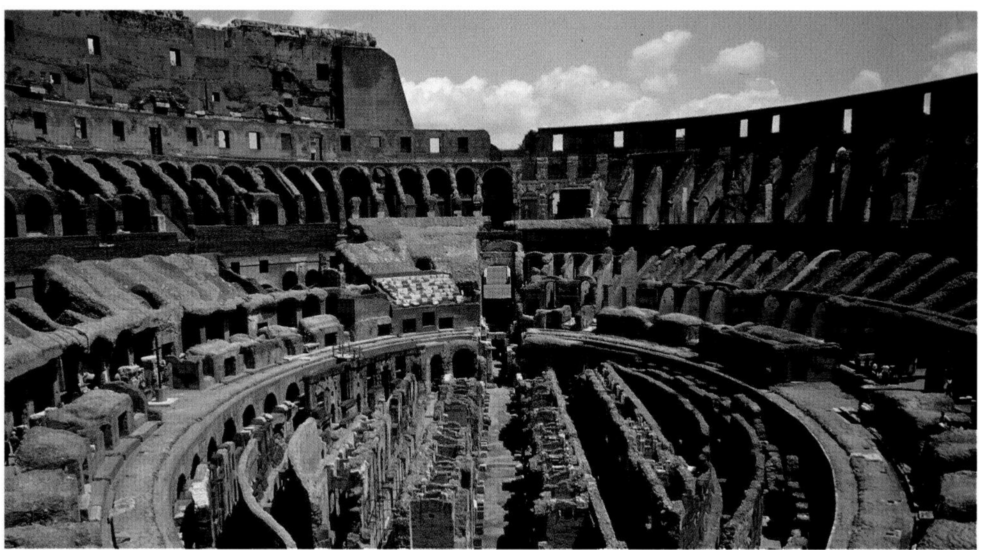

Water – the pride of Rome

Sextus Julius Frontinus was an engineer and water commissioner in Rome in 97 CE. Not surprisingly, he was very proud of Rome's engineering feats:

As a result of the increase in the number of works, reservoirs, fountains and water-basins, the air is purer; and the causes of the unwholesome atmosphere, which gave the city a bad name, are now removed. With such an array of indispensable structures carrying so much water, compare, if you will, the idle Pyramids or the useless, though famous, works of the Greeks.

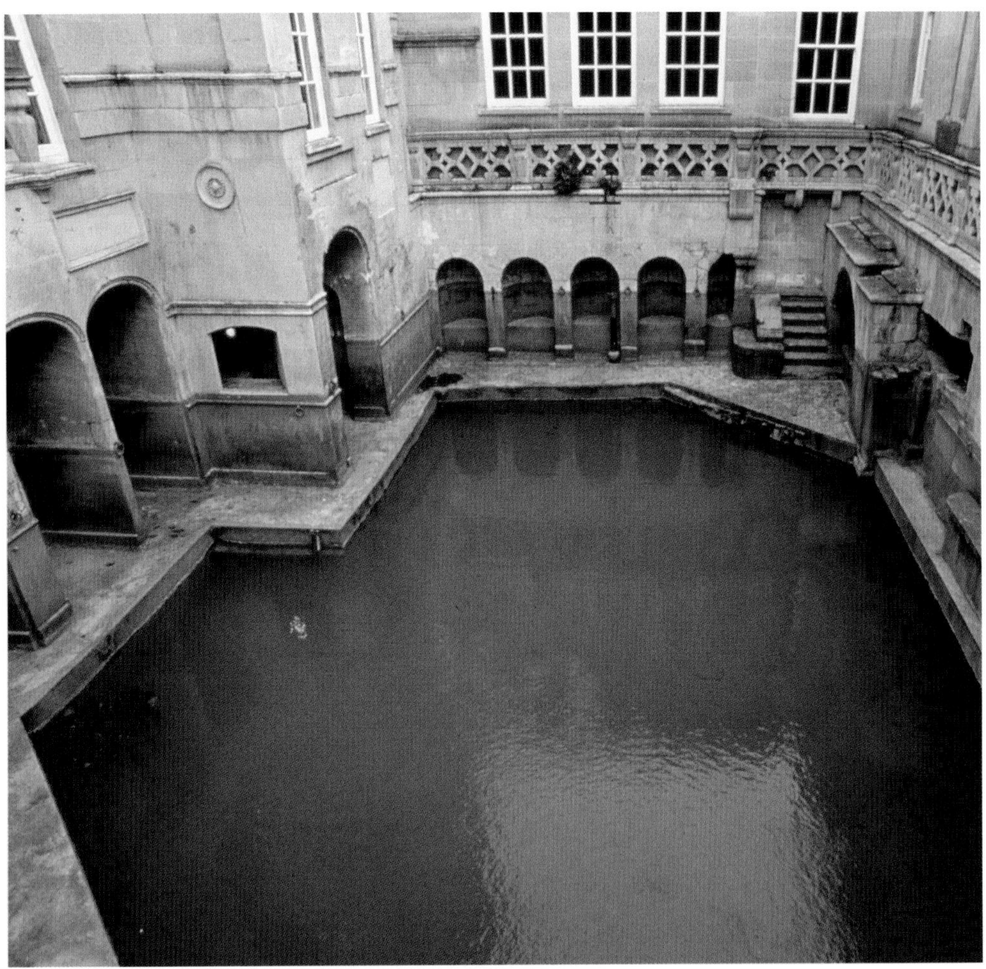

The Roman baths at Bath in southern England. Memorial stones show that legionaries came to Bath to drink the health-giving waters, convalesce and pray to the gods for a good recovery.

A visit to the baths

The Romans realized the importance of cleanliness for staying healthy. They built public baths in towns of all sizes and at military forts. The entrance fee was as low as possible, one quadrans (which was the smallest Roman coin), in order to encourage people to use the baths. By the end of the fourth century CE, there were 11 public baths and 926 private baths in Rome alone. The bath of Diocletian, built in 305 CE, could accommodate over 3000 bathers.

At the heart of the baths were the hot and cold plunge pools and steam rooms, where people could remove sweat and dirt with metal scrapers called *strigils*. However, the baths were much more than places to get clean. Baths were meeting places, where friends came to chat or gossip and where people came to do business, play ball games, exercise with a fitness coach or be pummelled by a masseur. Men, women and children used the baths but men and women bathed separately, women often using the baths early in the morning. Unfortunately, baths were also places where thieves had a good chance of stealing clothes and any valuables left lying around!

The cold room in the bath-house at Segedunum on Hadrian's Wall. This bath-house was recently reconstructed. It opened in 2000 to show people today how the Romans lived.

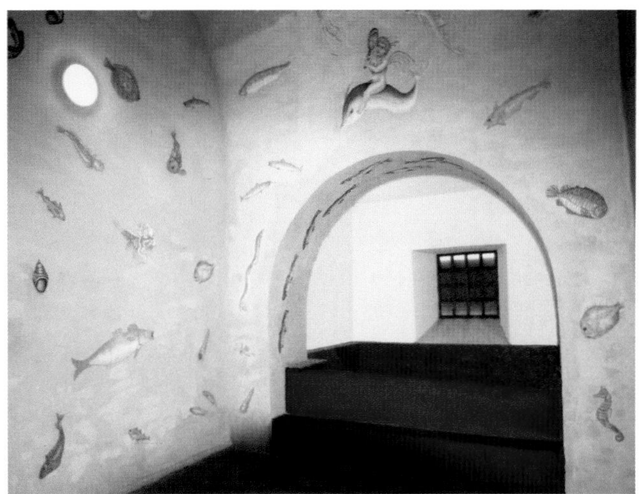

Even in Britain, on the edge of the Empire, baths were very popular. Archaeological excavations have shown that the baths in Wroxeter in Shropshire had an outdoor swimming pool and a massive exercise hall. Five hundred people a day probably used the baths in towns such as Wroxeter and Leicester. Five thousand people may have visited the baths each week in the larger city of Lincoln. This suggests a very clean and healthy population – except for one small problem. The water was only changed once a week!

The baths in Rome

Seneca was a Roman politician and writer who, around 50 CE, wrote a series of famous letters about life in Rome. Here is an extract from one letter:

In the early days there were few baths. People did not worry about the water being pure when they knew they were only going to make it dirty! Nevertheless, the local officials used to inspect these baths and make sure that they were kept clean and warm enough for comfort and health. But who nowadays could bear to bathe in such a fashion? We think ourselves poor if our walls are not covered with huge mirrors, if our ceilings are not buried in glass and our swimming pools lined with marble, and if the water does not pour out of silver spouts.

Very public toilets!

Good water supplies made public toilets possible. Earlier peoples had built public toilets but not on the same scale as the Romans. By 315 CE there were 144 public toilets in Rome, many situated in the baths, and they really were public. Individual cubicles were rare. Up to twenty people could be seated around three sides of a room. The latrines were flushed by mains water that had already been used in the baths.

Did the sewers help to keep people healthy?

Sewers were another great Roman engineering feat, but they were only successful if there was plenty of water and it was running swiftly enough to flush the sewage along. In York, for example, the sewers were simply too large and so the water did not flow through them quickly enough. The result was that sewage sat in the bottom of the sewers, especially when there was little rainfall. Another problem was that the rough surface of the stone sewers trapped the microbes that cause disease. A final danger was that sewers emptied into the local river, polluting the water that people drank or

The public latrines in the Roman town of Dougga in modern Tunisia, north Africa. They were built near the public baths. You can see the wash-basin on the right of the photograph.

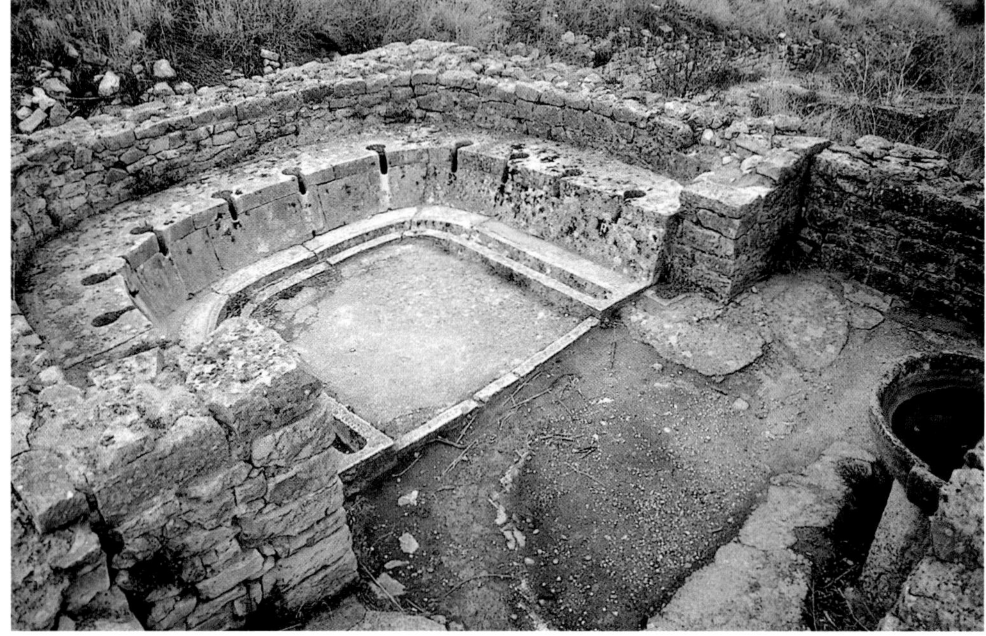

used for washing their clothes. The result was that the sewers of York actually contributed to the spread of disease, rather than preventing it. Cholera, an infectious disease spread by infected water, was rife in hot summers.

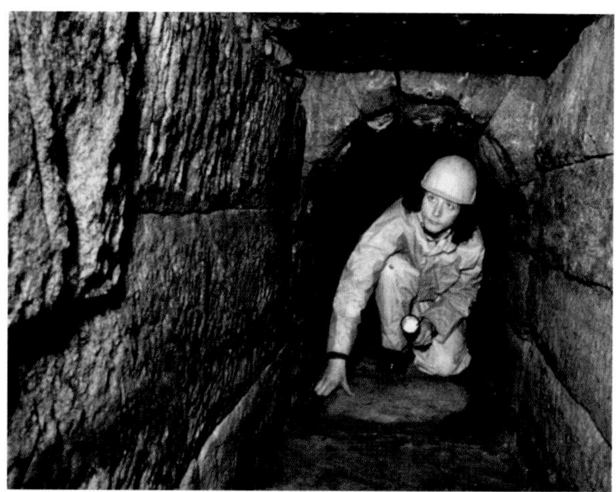

The Roman sewer in York. Manholes were built into the sewer to enable the channel to be cleaned out or checked for obstructions.

The Romans and the spread of disease

The Romans worked hard at preventing disease. They chose the sites of forts and towns carefully, provided clean water, built baths and sewers and employed engineers to look after their upkeep. Despite this, there were more outbreaks of epidemic disease during the time of the Roman Empire than before. This was not a coincidence. Legionaries, marching along those wonderful, straight roads, carried disease wherever they went. They first carried smallpox to Rome from the Middle East, causing an epidemic in 165 CE that killed around five million people. Sixty years later, there was another outbreak, killing 5000 people a day. Unfortunately the Romans were just as good at spreading diseases as they were at preventing them.

Death trap

There were dangers to health all around Rome. Many Romans lived in apartment blocks, but water supplies and sewers could only reach the ground floor. Residents had to carry their water upstairs and their solution to waste disposal was recorded by the poet Juvenal:

Along your route each open window may be a death trap. So hope and pray, poor man, that the local housewives drop nothing worse on your head than a bedpan full of slops!

Chapter 9

How successful was Greek and Roman medicine?

Greek and Roman doctors were handicapped, like all doctors before the 1860s, by not understanding that bacteria cause diseases. Hippocrates had put forward the first rational explanation for disease, but it was not correct. Ancient doctors also lacked the wide range of drugs and equipment that we take for granted today, such as antibiotics and thermometers. To the Greeks and Romans, even today's most everyday medical methods, such as X-rays, would seem miraculous gifts from the gods. Appendicitis, which today requires just a routine operation, was then always fatal.

Could Greek and Roman doctors help their patients?

Some of the simplest advice did make a difference. Doctors who advised their patients to eat a good diet and take plenty of exercise were helping them stay

Roman doctors had a difficult task advising their wealthy patients about the value of eating a good diet. The rich were used to lavish and exotic meals and plenty of alcohol, which sometimes led to heart attacks, liver problems and a range of other ailments. In this Roman mosaic the rich enjoy a lavish banquet on the banks of the River Nile.

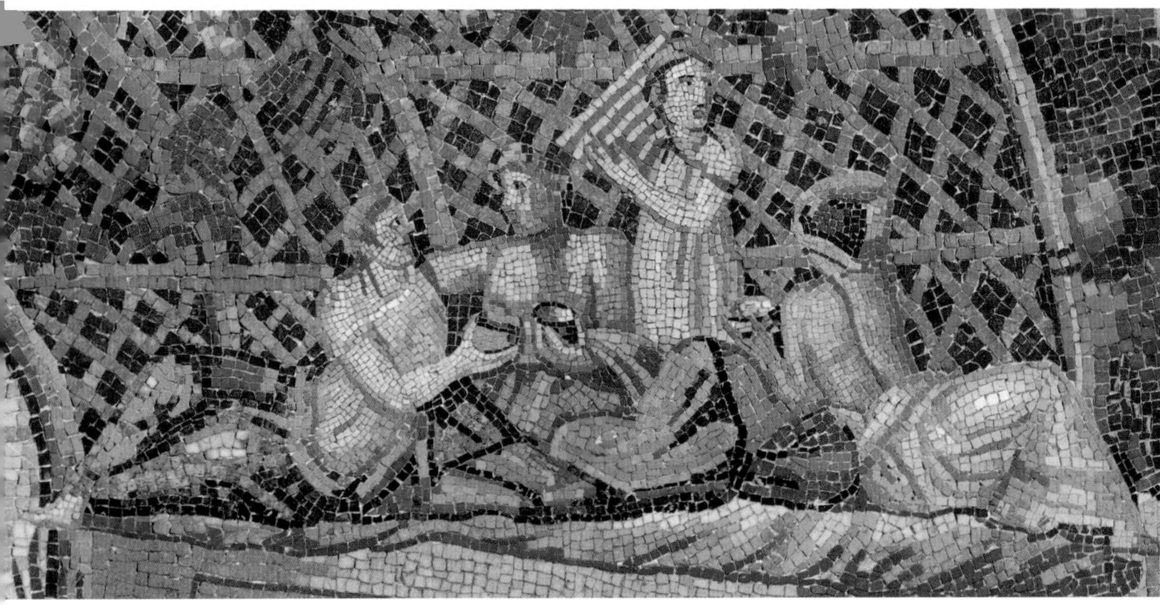

healthy and increasing their chances of recovery. The use of herbal remedies at all levels of society benefited many patients. Simple surgery, such as removing cataracts from eyes, was common and the surgeons developed considerable expertise by repeating the same basic operations. Many people would also have felt better because of their belief in their doctors or in the priests ministering to them at the temples of Asclepios.

Life expectancy

Although there is little evidence of life expectancy from the Greek Empire, Roman tombstones and skeletons give us a good indication of how long people lived at that time. This evidence suggests that 50 per cent of men had died by the age of 46 and 50 per cent of women by 34. However, ten per cent of Roman citizens did live to at least 65 and the rich, especially men, had as good a chance of living to be 70 as anyone born in the nineteenth century. We know from her tombstone, that one lady from Lincoln, Claudia Crysis, lived to be 90.

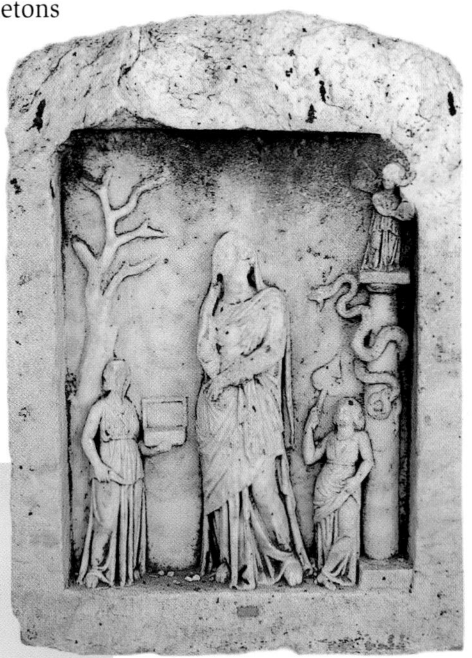

A Roman tombstone from the town of Izmir in modern Turkey. The dead woman (centre) is shown at the altar to Asclepios, whose sacred snake is shown on the right.

Tell-tale bones

What else can we learn from skeletons? Scientists examining bones have discovered the following information about the people of Roman Britain:

- Average height of men – 1.68 metres
- Average height of women – 1.55 metres
- They were strong and muscular, but 80 per cent of people suffered from osteo-arthritis, a painful swelling of the joints, caused by heavy, physical work, such as carrying water from wells to homes several times a day.
- They did not suffer from as much tooth decay as people today, but their teeth were very worn down by grains of stone in bread.

Medicine and a good story

In the adventure story *The Eagle of the Ninth* by Rosemary Sutcliff, Marcus, a young Roman soldier, sets out northwards across Hadrian's Wall to find the Eagle, the symbol carried proudly at the head of his father's legion, the Ninth. No one knows what has happened to the legion, but there are rumours that the eagle has been seen and will be used to rally the local tribes to rebel against Rome. How does the young soldier in this story travel unsuspected among hostile tribes? He disguises himself as a travelling eye-doctor!

The author based this part of her story on archaeological finds such as the eye-doctor's stamp pictured here.

Some healers specialized in treating eye infections, which were extremely common. This eye doctor's stamp gives his name, the name of the salve, or mixture, and what it was used to treat. The doctor made up the salve, rolled it like pastry into short lengths and stamped it with his name before using it.

The danger of giving birth

The difference between the life expectancies of men and women is largely the result of the dangers to women during childbirth. When archaeologists excavated a Roman cemetery at Poundbury in Dorset they found that eighteen per cent of the women buried there had died in or shortly after giving birth. This huge death toll is similar to evidence from other sites and is much the same as in the prehistoric period. Apart from the dangers from births not going to plan, women were at great risk from infections that could be passed on from unsterilized equipment, either from the midwife herself or from any of the other people who crowded round at the time of the birth. The newly born were also extremely vulnerable to infections. Around a quarter of Roman babies died before their first birthdays.

Prayer – the best remedy?

Generally doctors could help their patients with some health problems, but there were many more problems they could not cure. Even Galen admitted, "Confidence and hope do more good than medicines. The doctor is nature's assistant." It is little wonder that people continued to pray to their gods and visit the temples of Asclepios. Under the Romans, the new Christian church also insisted that the best cure for sickness was to pray and repent the sins that had caused the illness.

The end of the Roman Empire

The Roman Empire slowly collapsed in the fourth century when it was attacked by people the Romans called barbarians – the 'uncivilized' people living outside the Empire. The barbarians, the Goths and Vandals in central Europe and the Angles and Saxons in the west saw Roman villas and towns as treasure-houses simply waiting to be pillaged. Gradually, the Roman government withdrew its legions from the Empire to defend Rome itself from attacks, but this did not save Rome. It was attacked and looted by the Goths in 410 CE. The world that had enabled doctors to put forward new ideas and develop their treatments was dying rapidly.

In this nineteenth-century painting by Thomas Cole, the horror of the destruction of Rome is vividly portrayed.

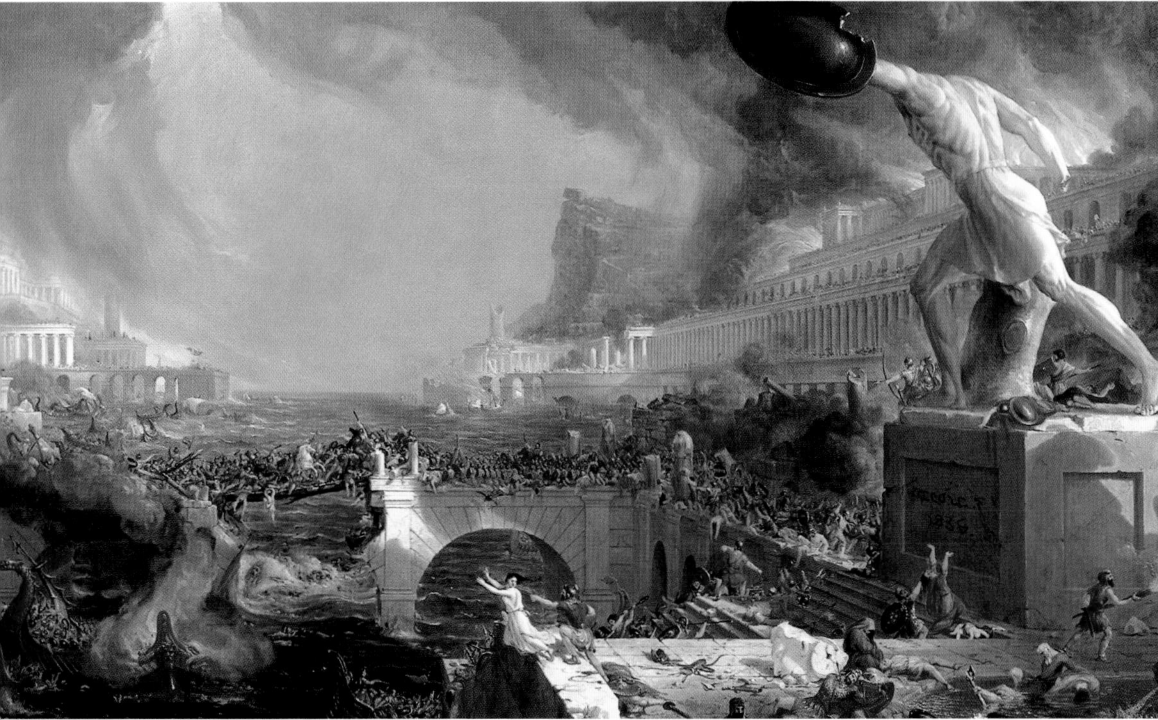

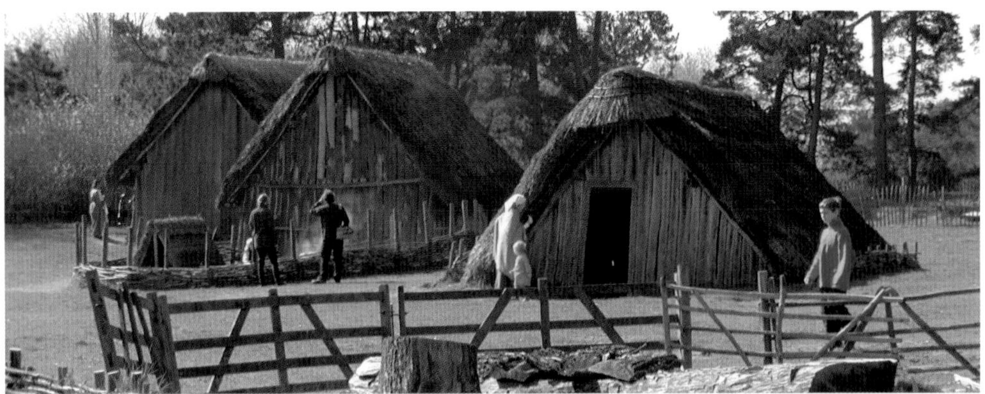

The Saxons who invaded Britain as the Roman Empire collapsed lived in homes like these reconstructed ones in West Stow, Sussex. Their homes and their medical treatments were very similar to those of the ordinary people in Roman Britain.

The future of medicine

Destruction and change had little impact on the medicine of ordinary people, the 90 per cent of the population who lived by farming. They had never known the names of Hippocrates or Galen. For them medicine continued to be provided, as it always had been, by the women of the household, whose wide-ranging knowledge of herbal remedies was passed down from mother to daughter.

Townspeople were more likely to be affected by the collapse of the Empire. There were no longer doctors in the towns. The baths, sewers and water supplies decayed as the towns themselves gradually disintegrated. The towns had grown wealthy on trade and some had grown up around legionary forts. Now there were no legions and there was no strong government to keep the peace and protect merchants as they travelled around the country. Entire Roman towns, such as Silchester in Hampshire, were deserted.

The survival of Hippocrates and Galen

Fire and looting destroyed many medical books. However, knowledge of Hippocrates, Galen and other doctors did survive. Medical writings and knowledge had been developing for more than 800 years and so was not easily wiped out. Some medical books survived in Christian monasteries and many more were preserved in Alexandria, the great centre of medical education for hundreds of years.

Another place of safety for the theories of Hippocrates and Galen was in the Arab world. Arab rulers in cities such as Baghdad and Damascus paid for Greek and Roman medical books to be translated into Arabic. Over time the Arab world became the springboard for Europe's own revival of interest in Hippocrates and Galen, in the theory of the Four Humours and treatments by opposites. In the eleventh and twelfth centuries, the Arabic texts were translated back into Latin and became the basis for medical studies in the new universities springing up in western Europe. The work of Hippocrates and Galen was about to flourish once more.

This wall painting in the cathedral of Anagni in Italy shows Galen (on the left) learning from Hippocrates. The painting dates from around 1250, showing how important Hippocrates and Galen still were over 800 years after the fall of the Roman Empire.

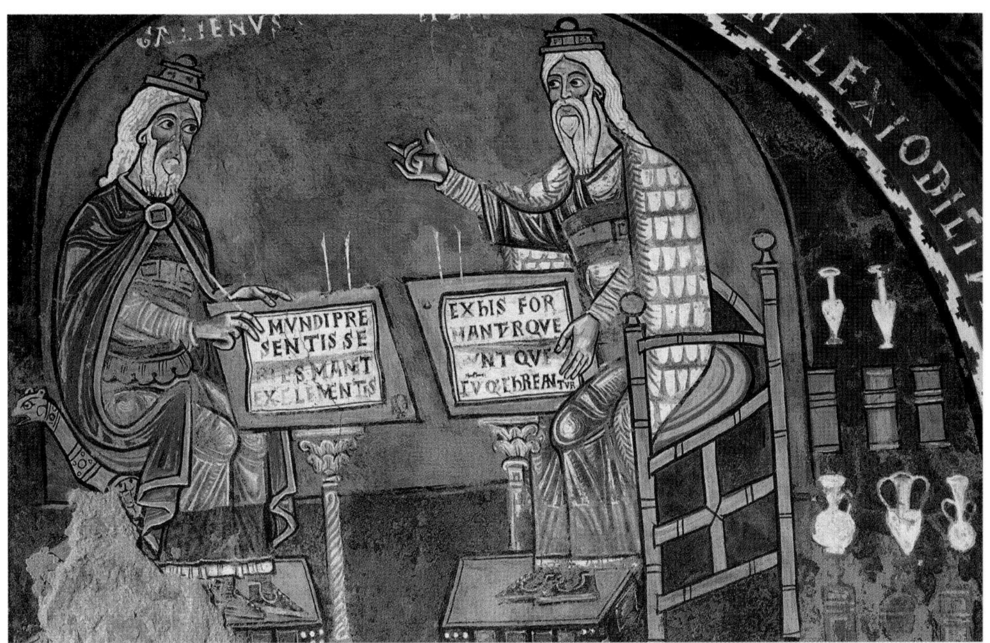

Some last advice from Galen!

For all his boasting, Galen did give his patients good advice. Here is one example:

Hunger is no reason for our greedily filling our bellies to excess, nor does it justify thirsting until the jug is emptied in one gulp. We must be careful to eat less than our guests, to refrain from delicacies and to eat sound food in moderate portions.

Glossary

Amulet a charm that the wearer believes gives protection from illness

Anaesthetic a drug that makes a person unconscious

Anatomy the study of the structure of the human body

Anoint to cover in oil as part of a ceremony or treatment

Antibiotic a drug used to treat infections caused by bacteria

Antiseptic a chemical or a natural substance that destroys bacteria and kills infection

Arteries the blood vessels that carry blood away from the heart

Bile a fluid created in the body that is sometimes vomited during illness

Cataract a growth on the eye that obscures vision

Choleric angry, irritated

Compendium a collection of information

Dissection the cutting up and scientific examination of human and animal bodies

Dysentery a severe illness causing frequent, fluid bowel movements

Embryo the unborn child or animal in the womb

Epidemic a disease affecting a large number of people at once

Epilepsy a nervous disease causing convulsions and loss of consciousness

Extremities the hands and feet

Fasting going without food

Fresco a painting on plaster, often on a wall

Gangrene the infection of dead human tissue, which can kill the victim unless the tissue is removed

Gladiators slaves and prisoners of war who were trained to fight each other or animals as public entertainment in Ancient Rome

Hemlock a poisonous plant and the drug obtained from the plant, sometimes used as an anaesthetic

Henbane a poisonous plant and the drug obtained from the plant, sometimes used as an anaesthetic

Homicide murder

Immunity protection against a disease

Inlaid decorative carving

Mandrake a poisonous plant and the drug obtained from the plant, sometimes used as an anaesthetic

Melancholic sad, gloomy

Midwife a woman who assists at a birth

Pestle and mortar a bowl and implement used to crush plants and other ingredients to make medicines

Pharmacy the study of drugs and how they are made for use as medicines

Phlegmatic sluggish, not easily excited

Physiology the study of how the body works

Pillage to plunder, rob

Pneumonia inflammation of the lungs due to infection

Purge to cleanse the body by taking drugs which make the drug-takers vomit or empty their bowels

Renaissance a period in European history from the fourteenth to the sixteenth centuries CE, when scientists and others were rediscovering what was learned in Ancient Greece and Rome and making many new discoveries

Sanguine optimistic, cheerful or of the colour of blood

Stadia a Greek measurement of distance. Ten stadia is around 1900 metres

Trepanning (also trephining) drilling a hole into the skull for medical reasons

Veins blood vessels that carry blood towards the heart

Votive stones carvings made to give thanks for recovery from illness

Timeline

Events		People
The first Olympic games **776**		
	500 BCE	
		Hippocrates born ***c.*** **470**
Plague of Athens **430–427**		
	400 BCE	
		Aristotle **384–322**
		Alexander the Great **356–323**
		Herophilus **335–280**
		Erasistratus ***c.*** **330–255**
	300 BCE	
Plague of Rome **295** – introduction of worship of Asclepios to Rome		
Roman army conquered all Italy **250**		
	200 BCE	
	100 BCE	Julius Caesar **100–44**
	BCE/CE	
		Celsus born ***c.*** **20**
		Pliny the Elder **23–79**
Building of the Roman baths at Bath – late first century CE		Roman conquest of Britain under Emperor Claudius **43**
		Dioscorides **40–90**
	100 CE	
c. **120 CE** Building of Hadrian's Wall; the period of the greatest extent of Roman Empire		Galen **131–200**
	200 CE	
	300 CE	
Building of baths of Diocletian **305**		
Pillage of Rome by barbarian tribes **410** and the Fall of the Roman Empire	**400 CE**	

Further information

Books

Blood and Guts, A Short History of Medicine,
Roy Porter, Penguin, 2002
An entertaining, up-to-date history for older readers.

Health and Medicine through Time,
Ian Dawson and Ian Coulson, John Murray, 1996
The most widely used schoolbook for examinations on this topic.

Ancient Greece and the Mediterranean,
Michael Kerrigan, BBC Books, 2001

Ancient Rome and the Mediterranean,
Michael Kerrigan, BBC Books, 2001
Two beautifully illustrated, clear histories of Greece and Rome for older readers.

The Rotten Romans,
Terry Deary, Scholastic Hippo, 1994

The Groovy Greeks,
Terry Deary, Scholastic Hippo, 1995
Entertaining, funny and informative.

Gods and Goddesses in Ancient Greece,
Peter Hicks, Hodder Wayland, 2002

History Beneath Your Feet Ancient Greece,
Fiona Macdonald, Hodder Wayland, 2003

Life in Roman Britain,
Tony McAleavy, English Heritage, 1999

Rome, Oxford University Press,
A. Solway and S. Biesty, 2003
A selection of well-illustrated information books on daily life and other key aspects of Roman and Greek history.

The Eagle of the Ninth, Oxford University Press,
Rosemary Sutcliff, 2000
A thrilling historical novel set in Roman Britain. Roman medicine plays an important part in the plot.

Websites

www.hadrians-wall.info
A guide to all the forts and sites on the Wall, plus information for visitors, such as places to stay.

www.museum.ncl.ac.uk
Run by the University of Newcastle, it includes Reticulum, the award-winning children's site on Ancient Rome.

www.vindolanda.com
A guide to the excavation of the Roman fort at Vindolanda on Hadrian's Wall, perhaps the most important archaeological excavation currently taking place in Britain.

www.archaeology.co.uk
Details of the magazines *Current Archaeology* and *Current World Archaeology* plus access to past editions.

www.julen.net/ancient
A really useful guide to a wide range of websites that deal with ancient history and archaeology.

www.spartacus.schoolnet.co.uk
A wide-ranging site that includes links to many sites covering ancient history.

www.bbc.co.uk/ancient
Entertaining information on the Greeks and Romans, plus activities and games.

www.english-heritage.org.uk
Information on Roman and other historical sites in Britain that are open to the public.

www.thebritishmuseum.ac.uk
Details and visuals of the museum's collections, which include many Greek and Roman objects.

www.medicalmuseums.org
A guide to ten medical museums in and around London.

Places to visit

Thackray Medical Museum, Beckett Street, Leeds
Interactive displays on the history of medicine, designed for all ages.
www.thackraymuseum.org.uk

The Science Museum, London
Displays on many aspects of science, including medicine.
www.sciencemuseum.org.uk

Segedunum Roman Fort, Baths and Museum, Wallsend, Newcastle
The reconstructed bath-house at Segedunum near Newcastle.
www.segedunum.com

The Roman Baths, Bath
Audio-tour of the excavated site.
www.romanbaths.co.uk

Index